CW00925102

MY HAPPY PREGNANCY COOK BOOK

Copyright 2016 Emma Thomson

The rights of Emma Thomson to be identified as the author of this work has been asserted by her in accordance with the Copyright, Designs and Patents Act.

All rights reserved. No part of this publication may be reproduced, stored in a retrieval system or transmitted, in any form or by any means, without the prior consent of the author, or be otherwise circulated in any form of binding or cover other than that in which it is published and without a similar condition being imposed on the subsequent purchaser.

Introduction

Pregnancy is such a unique and wonderful time that it should be celebrated. One of the key ways to enhance your journey is to really enjoy the food that you are eating. Great food should not only taste good, but should also give you the nutrients you need. Food and eating during pregnancy has unfortunately become associated with guilt, worry and anxiety. There is no need for this. My book shows you how to make eating great food a pleasurable experience that is good for your mind, body and of course your baby.

During my three pregnancies I found it very stressful working out what to eat and what not to eat. The rules and guidelines changed all the time. It was made even harder by knowing friends from other cultures who got different advice. All very confusing! Food certainly wasn't considered a pleasurable part of pregnancy. It was more about making me feel guilty for enjoying tasty food. Was I eating the right things? Or was I eating the wrong things that could affect my baby? Because I love food and cooking this was horrible for me. It also led to lots of anxious feelings when I had a treat or overindulged in something nice but a little bit naughty.

Researching for this book sadly proved the same thinking prevails today - eating during pregnancy is something very serious and not much fun at all. Eating good food is an important part of our lives. Being pregnant is a unique and special time and putting them together should create a great experience. That's why I simply had to write this book. I worked hard to keep it simple; you don't need to be a skilled chef to prepare the dishes, the recipes are quick and easy to cook and contain simple ingredients available from any supermarket. I've also made sure they are safe to eat in pregnancy, so you can relax and enjoy a mixture of healthy, nutritious and a little bit naughty food.

These recipes are not written as a strict plan to follow; they are intended to offer fun cooking ideas to help you create wonderful, happy memories of your pregnancy journey through sharing the joy of food and eating.

Contents

YOU ARE

Amazing

Wow, you are amazing! Stop and think about it for a moment, you are growing a brand new human being inside you! Your wellbeing is of the utmost importance at this time. Eating well is key to taking care of yourself and your baby. Even on the days when you feel tired, achy, nauseous or emotional, you should make time to celebrate the wonderful job that your body is doing. Take time to love yourself from the inside out and your baby will feel this emotion too.

Treat yourself to a pregnancy massage. Massage during pregnancy helps promote a good labour experience. You should work with a therapist who is qualified in pregnancy massage. Ask for vouchers for your birthday or Christmas. Your friends and family will want to support you and this lets them participate. You'll typically feel best during the middle three months of your term so this is a great time for you to go. Even when your bump is quite large, you will be able to use a pregnancy massage table or you can sit up and lean over the back of a chair with lots of cushions.

Alternatively, run a warm bath with your favourite bubbles and make time to relax. Light a candle, lie back and breathe deeply to let go of any tension. Spend a few minutes thinking about your baby. Stroke your tummy and speak softly. When you feel calm and relaxed, your baby will enjoy that feeling too. *Remember, you're so worth it.* ☺

'Feel Good' ASPARAGUS AND SPINACH SOUP

INGREDIENTS

1 tablespoon olive oil

250g fresh asparagus spears, stalks trimmed and cut up

2 shallots, finely chopped

1 garlic clove, crushed

2 large handfuls spinach

400mls vegetable stock

Makes 2 servings
Ready within 30 mins

This vibrant green, tasty soup is very quick and easy to make when you want something healthy without too much hassle. Both asparagus and spinach are packed full of folate which is an essential vitamin during your pregnancy for the prevention of neural tube defects. In the early months of pregnancy, you may find yourself suffering from regular snack attacks. This soup is a great snack option as it can be made quickly or reheated in minutes if made in advance. It is just as good a recipe made with tinned asparagus and frozen spinach meaning you can make this soup anytime of the year.

METHOD

1. Heat the oil in a pan and add the shallots, asparagus and garlic. Cook for 5 to 10 mins until softened.

2. Add the stock and bring up to a simmer. Cook for 5 mins until asparagus is tender.

3. Turn off the heat and stir through the spinach leaves.

4. Whizz the soup to a smooth consistency with a hand blender or food processor.

5. Return to the pan, season to taste and warm through before serving.

Delicious served with your favourite bread.

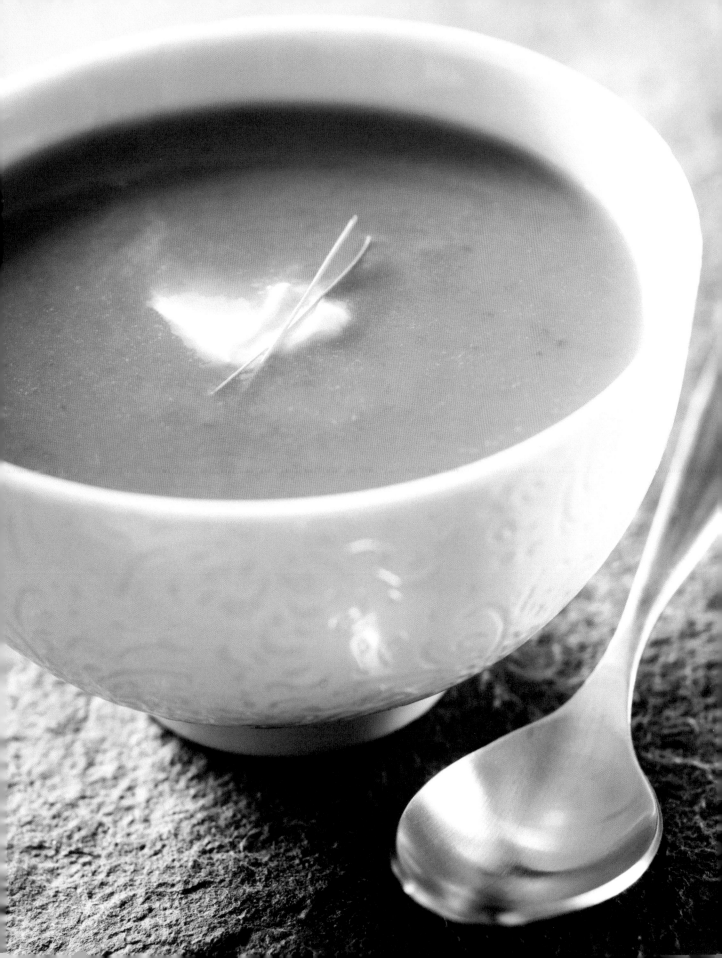

'Easy' STUFFED ROAST PEPPERS

INGREDIENTS

Olive oil

1 small onion, chopped

1 clove garlic, crushed

250g lean beef mince

1 can chopped tomatoes

2 teaspoons dried oregano

1 tablespoons tomato puree

1 teaspoon Worcester sauce

2 peppers (red or orange)

50g grated cheddar cheese

Serves 2
Preparation time 10 mins
Cooking time 45 mins

This easy supper dish is a nice treat after a long day at work. Choose lean beef mince which will provide less fat but all the benefits of protein and iron which are essential for your health and your baby's development.

Red peppers and tomatoes are full of vitamins and also lycopene which is a great antioxidant. These would also make a nice dish to take to work for a leftover lunch.

METHOD

1. Preheat oven to 200C (180 C fan).

2. Add the mince to a pan and turn up the heat. Cook the mince until it is browned all over.

3. Add the onion, garlic, oregano, tomato puree, tinned tomatoes and Worcester sauce and stir well.

4. Bring to the boil then reduce heat to a simmer. Cook for about 30 minutes until onion and beef are tender.

5. While mince is cooking, prepare the peppers. Cut them in half (through the stalk to form boat shapes) and remove the seeds.

6. Place the peppers in an oven proof dish, cut side up, and bake in the oven for 20 mins.

7. When the mince is cooked, divide it between the peppers (excess sauce can be frozen for another meal or served alongside).

8. Sprinkle over the cheese and return to the over for 10 mins until cheese is melted.

These can be served on their own or go well with wholegrain rice or pasta for added energy.

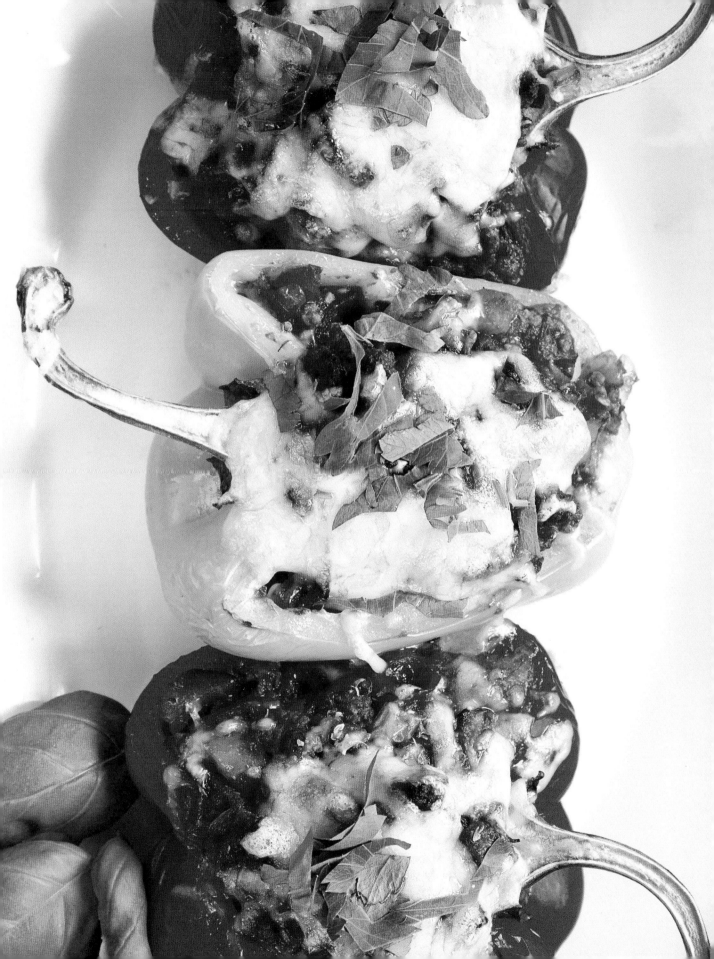

'Half way there' WARM LAMB WITH ROASTED VEG SALAD

INGREDIENTS

2 lamb steaks

1 small butternut squash (approx. 250g), peeled and seeds removed

1 courgette

1 red pepper

1 teaspoon dried thyme

1 tablespoon honey

Juice of half a lemon

100g baby spinach leaves

100g feta cheese, crumbled

Olive oil as required

Serves 2
Preparation time 10 mins
Cooking time 35 mins

Celebrate being half way through your pregnancy (around 20 weeks) with this delicious dish. You are likely to be feeling less tired now and beginning to enjoy the 'blooming' stage. You'll begin to feel your baby moving and have a small bump which looks like a real baby bump rather than a food baby. Keep looking after yourself as your new arrival will be here in less than 5 months.

METHOD

1. Preheat your oven to 200C (Fan 180C).

2. Cut up the squash, pepper and courgette in to bite size pieces and place in a large roasting tin. Add the thyme and olive oil and mix together well.

3. Put tin in the oven and roast for 15 mins.

4. Prepare lamb by rubbing a teaspoon of olive oil on both sides of each steak. Heat a non-stick frying pan and cook the lamb on both sides for about 15 mins until cooked through.

5. Meanwhile, take the vegetables out of the oven and mix in the honey and lemon juice. Return to the oven for another 10 mins or until veg are cooked through.

6. Transfer the cooked lamb to a clean board and allow to rest for a few minutes.

7. Remove the roasting tin from the oven and place on a heat resistant surface. Add the spinach leaves to the roasting tin with the feta cheese and mix everything together gently.

8. Slice the lamb on the board.

9. Serve by placing a portion of the roasted veg and feta on to a plate and topping with the sliced lamb.

Smile and remember the day that you will be meeting your baby for the first time is getting closer.

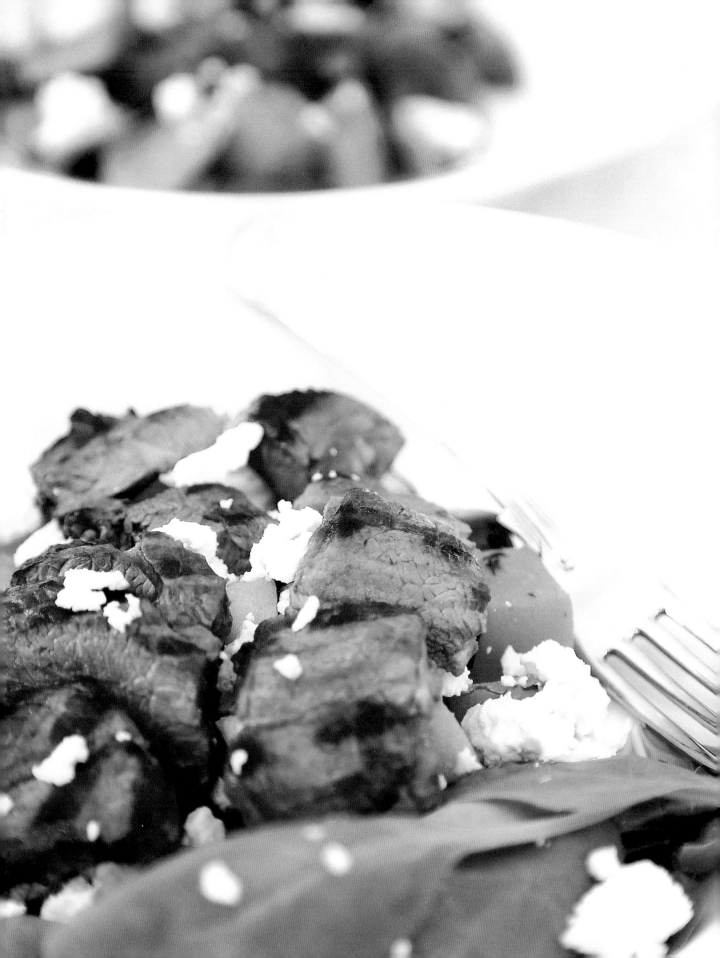

'Happy hormone'
NUTTY BROWNIES

INGREDIENTS

200g butter

200g good quality dark chocolate

300g caster sugar

4 medium eggs, lightly beaten

2 teaspoons vanilla extract

100g plain flour

50g cocoa powder

150g nuts such as hazelnuts, walnuts or pecans

Makes approx. 16 squares
Preparation time 15 mins
Cooking time 40 mins

It's a big day. You have your first appointment with your midwife. You may hear your baby's heartbeat for the first time or find out when your baby is due if you don't already know. Celebrate this exciting occasion by treating yourself (and your baby) to one of these very indulgent brownies. While you smile and take pleasure in eating, your body produces hormones which pass through your placenta to your baby. He or she will then also enjoy this feeling of pleasure and happiness from you. This is not an excuse to eat more though. One brownie is definitely enough. ☺

METHOD

1. Preheat oven to 180C (160C fan).

2. Put the nuts on a baking sheet and put in the oven to toast for approximately 10 minutes until light golden. Remove from oven and allow to cool for a few minutes.

3. Grease a 20 cm tin and line with baking parchment.

4. Put butter and chocolate in a large non-metallic bowl and melt in the microwave in 30 sec blasts, stirring in between. Once fully melted, gently combine and leave to cool for a few minutes.

5. Next add the sugar, eggs and vanilla to the melted chocolate and beat well with a wooden spoon.

6. Now add the flour and cocoa powder and stir to combine.

7. Finally add the toasted nuts and mix together.

8. Put the brownie mix in to the prepared tin and bake for 40 minutes.

9. Allow to fully cool in the tin (overnight in the fridge is good) before cutting in to squares.

Serve with your favourite cuppa or warm a brownie and eat as a dessert with cream or ice-cream. Bliss.

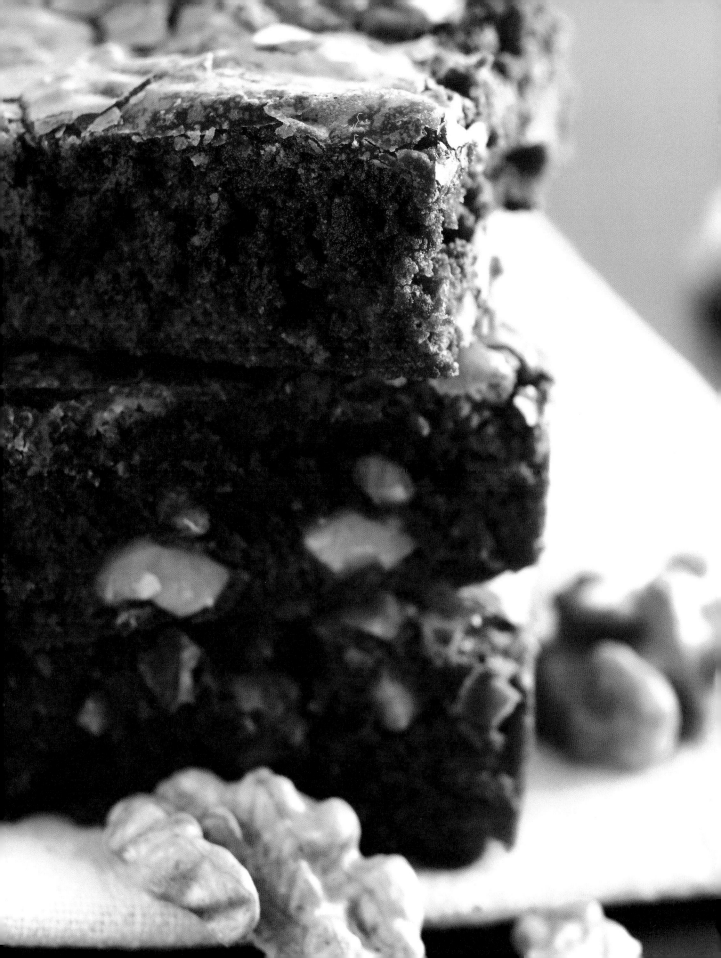

BANANA AND WALNUT LOAF

INGREDIENTS

125g butter

165g caster sugar

1 teaspoon vanilla

2 eggs

2 large or 3 small bananas, mashed

100g plain flour

100g self-raising flour

100g chopped walnuts

Makes approx. 12 slices
Preparation time 15 mins
Cooking time 45 mins

We know bananas are great for giving us slow release energy and are full of essential vitamins and minerals. They are a healthy choice throughout your pregnancy and this recipe is a good way for you to use up any over ripe bananas.

Take fifteen minutes to slow down and let any stress subside. Reflect on some of your best and happiest memories. Now that your relaxed, enjoy a slice of banana and walnut loaf with a cup of tea (in your favourite mug). You know you're worth it.

METHOD

1. Preheat oven to 200C (180C fan).

2. Grease and line a 700g or 7cm x 21cm loaf tin.

3. Beat butter, sugar and vanilla together with an electric mixer until light and fluffy.

4. Add eggs one at a time and beat to combine.

5. Stir in half the dry ingredients with half the bananas and stir to combine. Repeat with remaining flour and bananas.

6. Mix in the walnuts.

7. Carefully spoon the mixture in to the tin and bake for about 40 mins.

8. When the cake is ready, a skewer should come out clean when tested. (If the cake needs longer but is colouring too much on top, cover with tinfoil and return to the oven.)

9. Remove from oven and cool on a rack.

This cake should last for about 4 days in an airtight container but is unlikely to last that long. ☺

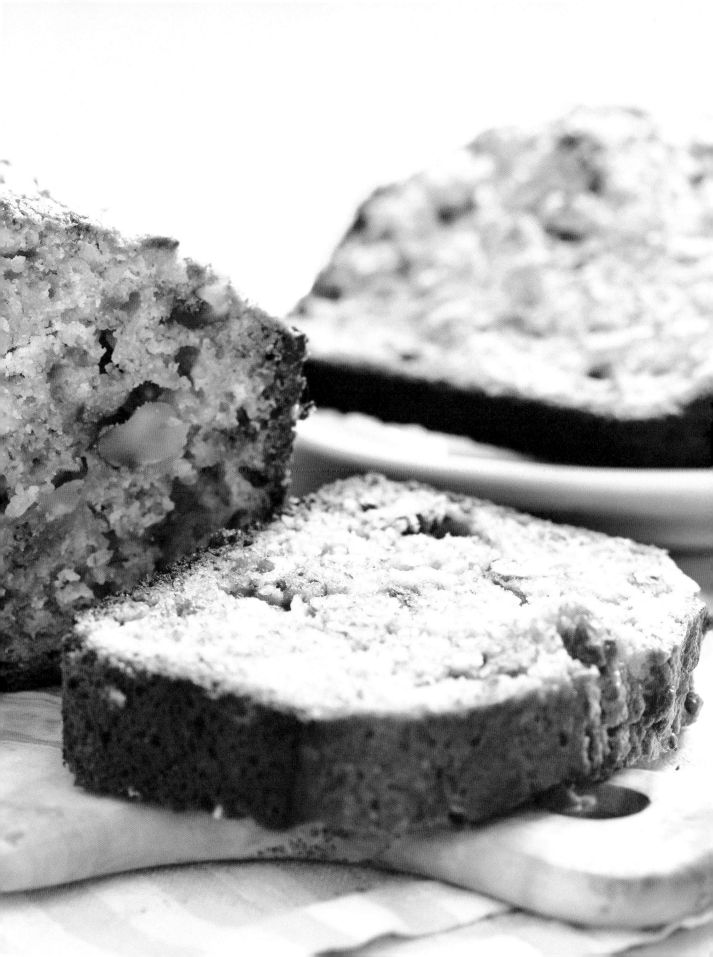

BREAKFAST, BRUNCHES &

Lie In's

You are a beautiful baby making goddess who needs lots of pampering and rest. Tiredness is common right through pregnancy although the first and last three months are notoriously the key 'tired trimesters'. If you are working full time, it can be difficult to get all the rest you need through the week so you should take the chance to nap whenever you can. A lie in on a Saturday or Sunday is a great way to get some extra sleep. Why not make it really special and have breakfast in bed? If you are lucky enough to have a partner who wants to spoil you, then show them these recipes and tips below and wait to be adored with food gifts on a tray. Alternatively, you can make yourself a lovely breakfast and head back to bed with a favourite magazine or book for an hour or so. Enjoy.

'Celebration' PANCAKES WITH MAPLE SYRUP AND WALNUTS

INGREDIENTS

100g walnut pieces

250g plain flour

1 tablespoon caster sugar

2 teaspoons baking powder

Pinch of salt

1 egg

250mls milk

2 tablespoons vegetable oil (plus more for cooking)

2 ripe bananas, mashed

½ teaspoon vanilla

100mls double cream (optional)

Maple syrup (to your taste)

Serves 3 hungry people (or 1 pregnant lady and her partner ☺)
Preparation time 10 mins
Cooking time 20 mins

These truly yummy pancakes are likely to become a future family favourite. They are a perfect start to an important day like a birthday, anniversary or just because you are loving life. Although they are a treat, they contain bananas which are a great source of potassium, essential to help manage your blood pressure effectively. The walnuts also contain a source of good fat needed by your growing baby. Why not plan these celebration pancakes for your first breakfast when you come home with your new baby and make it really memorable?

METHOD

1. If using walnuts, toast them lightly in the oven for an extra nutty flavour. Do this by heating your oven to 180C (160C fan). Place walnuts on a baking tray and pop in the oven to toast for about 10 mins. (Keep an eye on them as they burn easily).

2. Meanwhile, mix the flour, sugar, baking powder and salt in a bowl.

3. Put the milk in a separate bowl and add the egg. Beat lightly, then add oil, vanilla and bananas. Mix together.

4. Add banana mixture to flour mixture and mix gently.

5. Heat a lightly oiled frying pan over a medium heat. Using a small cup or ice cream scoop, place the pancake mixture in the pan. (3 pancake scoops at a time works well). Wait until small bubbles appear on the top of the pancake mixture before turning. Each side should be a golden brown colour. Keep these pancakes warm in a low oven and continue until all the mixture is used.

6. While waiting for pancakes to cook, pour the double cream in to a small bowl and using either an electric mixer or hand whisk, gently beat until the cream is thickened to your liking. (This is a great time to practice your pelvic floor exercises. While beating the cream, stand with your legs hip width apart, feet firmly on the floor. Relax your shoulders. Gently pull in your pelvic floor muscles and then relax them. Repeat this 10 times. For more information on the benefits of pelvic floor exercises, go to NHS Choices website).

To serve, place 2 or 3 overlapping pancakes on a warm plate. Put a dollop of cream on the top and scatter over the toasted nuts. Finish with a drizzle of maple syrup. Serve with a big smile and a toned pelvic floor.

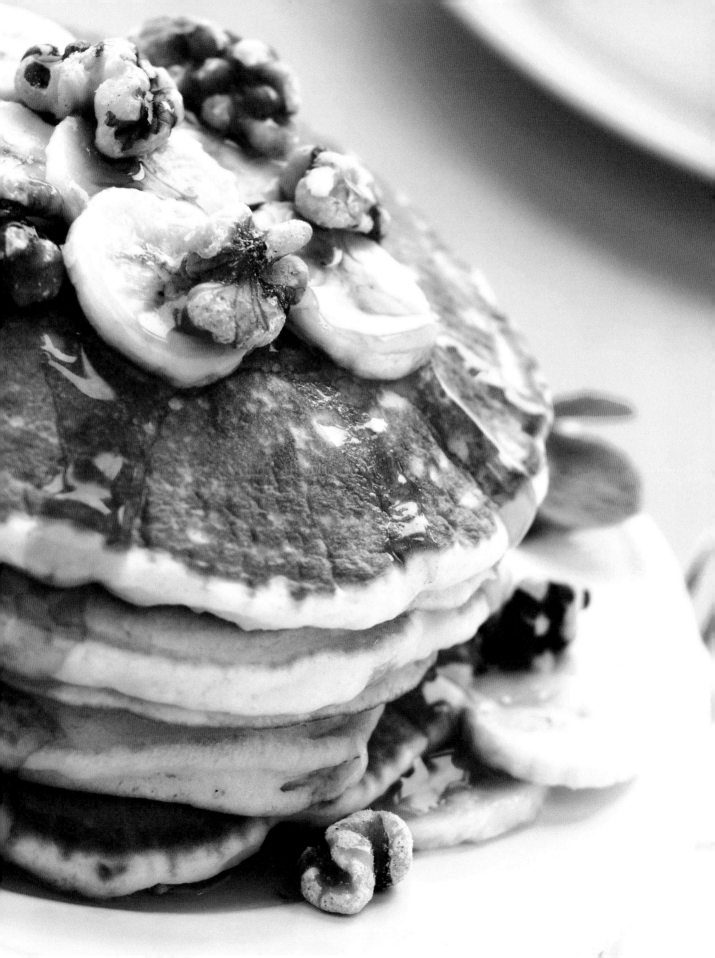

'Me time' MUESLI AND BLUEBERRY BREAD

INGREDIENTS

350g self-raising flour

50g muesli (your homemade pimped up muesli would work perfectly)

50g caster sugar

225 mls milk

25g butter, melted

1 egg, lightly beaten

175g blueberries

Makes approx. 12 slices
Preparation time 15 mins
Cooking time 45 mins

This bread is really delicious and not just for breakfast. It's a great snack at any time of the day. It tastes divine straight from the oven, warm with butter or sliced and toasted. It's nice to eat when you are not in a hurry and can enjoy it with your favourite cuppa. Have you thought about keeping a diary of your pregnancy? It can be a helpful way to address your hopes and fears for your future as a parent. It is also a wonderful record of all the exciting milestones of your pregnancy. Your child will love to read your diary in the future too. Why not buy a really pretty notebook and take time to write down your thoughts and feelings? Eating your lovely homemade blueberry bread while you write will make this time even more special.

METHOD

1. Preheat oven to 180C (170C fan).

2. Grease and line a 700g or 7cm x 21cm loaf tin. (Bought loaf tin liners are easiest).

3. Mix together the flour, muesli and sugar in a large bowl.

4. Make a well in the centre of the bowl and pour in the milk, eggs and butter.

5. Mix until combined and then add the blueberries. Mix again gently until blueberries are combined but not broken.

6. Pour mixture in to the tin and level the top.

7. Bake for 30 mins, then cover with foil and bake for a further 15 minutes.

8. The bread is ready when a cake tester comes out clean.

9. Cool on a wire rack.

To serve, cut carefully while still warm and spread with butter. Sit down, relax and enjoy. ☺

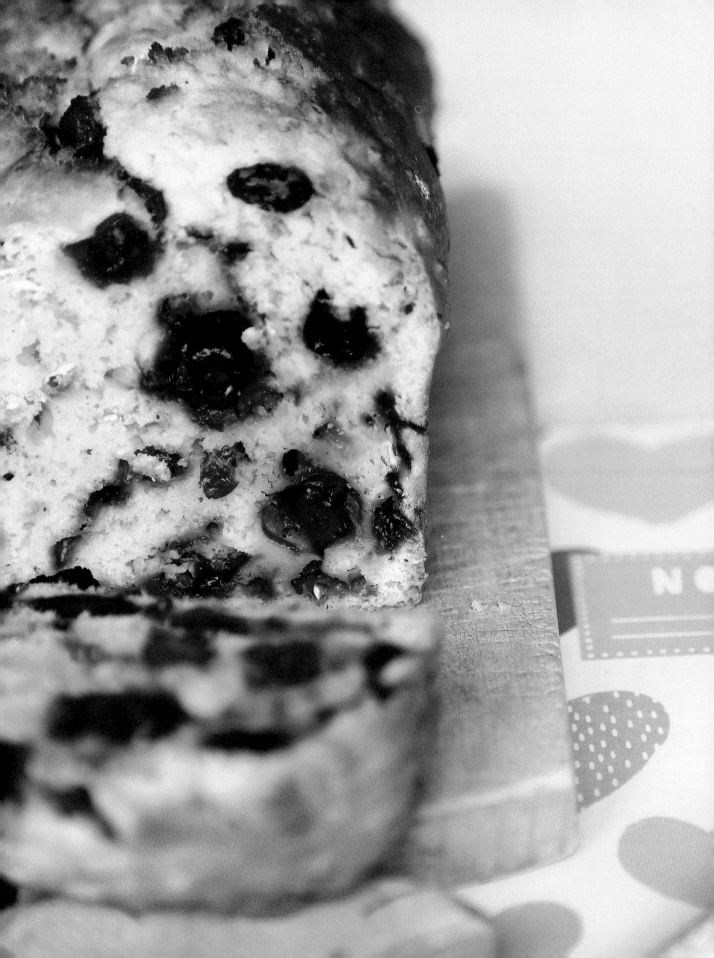

VANILLA OVERNIGHT OATS

INGREDIENTS

125g oats

170 mls water

*125mls low fat
vanilla yoghurt*

*1 tablespoon flaxmeal (or
crush some flax seeds yourself
in a mortar and pestle)*

*Berries, nuts, honey, maple
syrup or brown sugar for
toppings. Or any of your
other favourites.*

Serves 1
Preparation time 5 mins

These overnight oats take the hassle out of breakfast preparation because you make them the night before. Even if you have been struggling with tiredness in the mornings, there is one less thing to do when you get up. Although growing a baby is generally hard work and quite a tiring business, there are things that can lessen fatigue. Good iron levels can combat tiredness so make sure you include iron rich foods in your diet. The flaxseeds in this recipe are a good source of iron. Try almonds and chopped apricots as an alternative which provide iron too.

METHOD

1. Except for the toppings, place the ingredients (in order) in to a bowl. Don't stir.

2. Leave overnight in the fridge.

3. In the morning, stir the oat mixture and add your favourite toppings.

Feel on top of the world. ☺

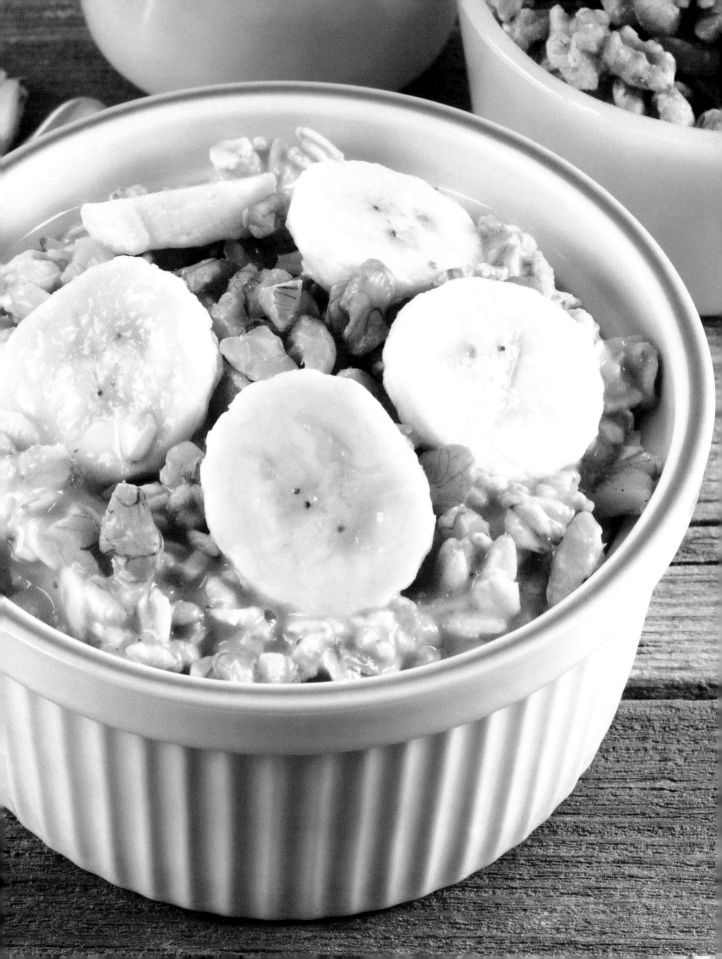

'Pimped up' MUESLI (OR BABY GRANOLA)

INGREDIENTS

2 tablespoons vegetable oil

125mls maple syrup

2 tablespoons honey

1 teaspoon vanilla extract

300g porridge oats

50g sunflower seeds

50g pumpkin seeds

2 tablespoons sesame seeds

2 tablespoons flaxseeds

50g flaked almonds

50g other nuts such as hazelnuts or pecans (add more nuts here if you like)

100g dried fruit such as apricots, sultanas or cranberries (add more fruit here if you want)

50g desiccated coconut (optional)

Makes 10 - 12 servings
Preparation time 10 mins
Cooking time 30 mins

Start your day with this delicious muesli-come-granola and you will be ready for anything. Even if you are not a big breakfast person, you can tailor make this recipe to suit your preferences, making it much more enjoyable. Pimp it up with yoghurt and berries or chopped fruit of your choice and you will never skip breakfast again.

METHOD

1. Heat oven to 150C (140C fan).

2. Mix the oil, syrup, honey and vanilla together in a large bowl.

3. Add the remaining ingredients to the bowl, except the dried fruit and coconut (if using).

4. Tip the granola mix out on to one large or two smaller baking sheets and spread out evenly.

5. Bake for 15 mins.

6. Remove from the oven and mix in the fruit and coconut. Return to the oven for a further 15 mins.

7. Remove from the oven and allow to cool fully before tipping in to an airtight container to store.

Best served with natural yoghurt and your favourite mix of chopped fruit or berries. Also great as a bedtime snack served simply with milk.

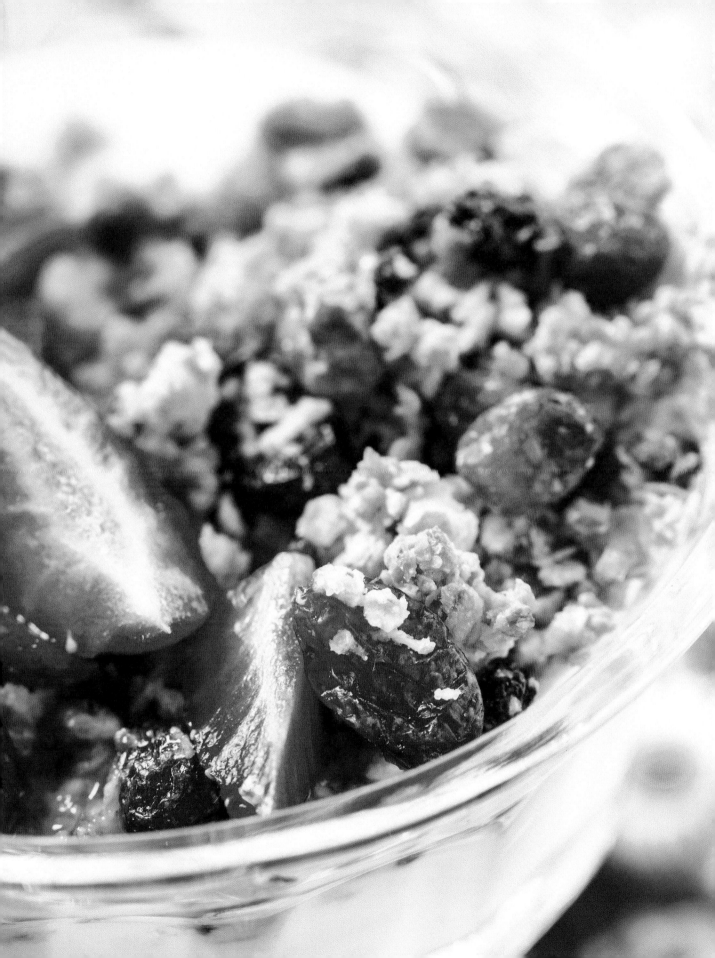

'Stomach settling'
GINGER BISCUITS

INGREDIENTS

150g self-raising flour

75g sugar

2 teaspoons ground ginger

1 teaspoon bicarbonate of soda

100g butter

1 tablespoon syrup

2 pieces of stem ginger, finely chopped (optional)

Makes approx. 15 biscuits
Preparation time 10 mins
Cooking time 20 mins

Ginger is commonly known to ease symptoms of nausea and help settle an unhappy tummy. These little biscuits are super quick to make and are easy to nibble when you are feeling queasy. If you are suffering from morning sickness, keep a few by your bed to eat when you first waken. For all day sickness, keep some in your handbag and at your desk at work to alleviate those stomach churning moments. Eating little and often is a good tip for reducing sickness.

METHOD

1. Preheat oven to 170C (150C fan).

2. Line a baking tray with parchment or lightly grease with butter.

3. Mix dry ingredients together in a bowl.

4. Melt syrup and butter gently in a pan. Add to dry ingredients and mix well. Add the stem ginger and mix – if using.

5. Place walnut size pieces on the baking tray a little apart.

6. Press them down with the back of a fork.

7. Bake in the oven for 15 to 20 mins until they are a pale golden brown.

8. Allow to cool for 5 mins before transferring to a rack to cool completely.

9. Store in an airtight container.

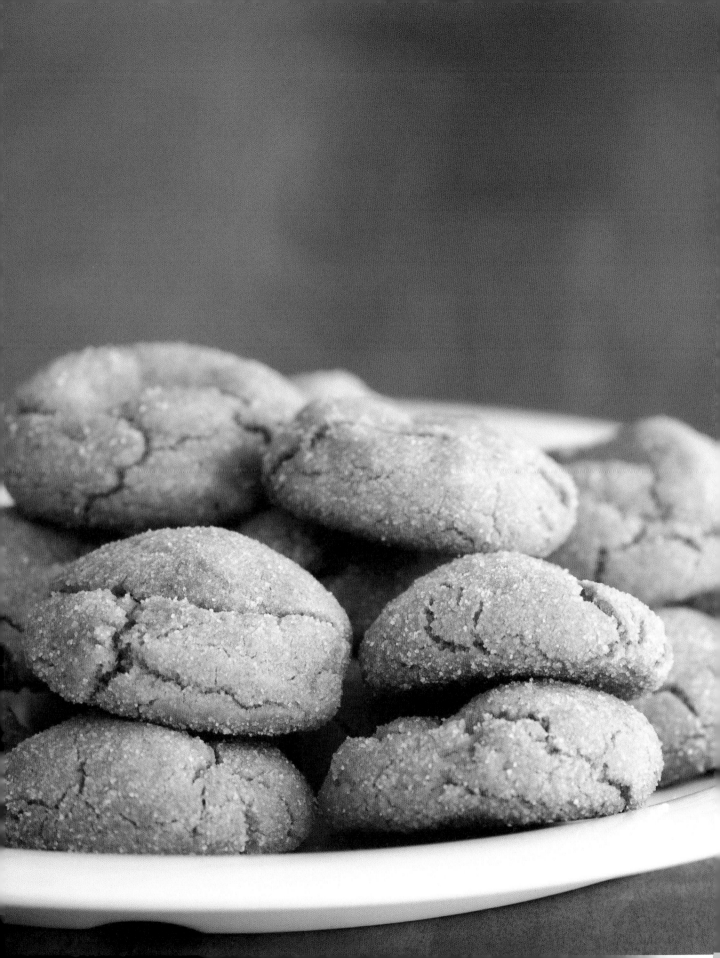

WORKING
Lunches

Working whilst you are pregnant can be challenging in lots of ways. It's also easy to believe that being at work means that you can't keep fit and healthy or make the time to celebrate being pregnant. The good news is that you can achieve all these things but you need to be organised and plan ahead.

A good way is to make the most of your work break times (you are legally entitled to these). If possible, get away from your workstation to eat. Plan what you will eat in advance so that you have something to look forward to. This helps break up your work day too. Take time to eat and enjoy your meal. If possible, have a walk in the fresh air after eating allowing you to begin work again feeling refreshed. A walk can also help if you suffer from an 'after lunch' slump. If you feel really exhausted, take a power nap in your pregnancy rest area (all employers should provide somewhere for a pregnant employee to rest even if it is just a quiet area). It might feel a bit cheeky but much better to have a rest and then be productive in your role than spend the whole afternoon pinching yourself to stay awake. It's much safer for you and your baby too.

'Sunshine in a bowl'
TOMATO AND LENTIL SOUP

INGREDIENTS

Olive oil

1 onion, chopped

1 clove of garlic, chopped

180g red lentils

1 can chopped tomatoes

1 litre of vegetable stock

1 tablespoon fresh coriander, chopped

1 teaspoon turmeric

Half teaspoon paprika

Makes 6 servings
Preparation time 10 mins
Cooking time 40 mins

This healthy and hearty soup is great for chasing away the hunger pangs at lunch time. It's full of lentils which are a great source of protein and essential for your baby's growth. Tomatoes provide lots of vitamins and minerals and certainly count as one of you five a day. What more could you want? Eat this soup with a hunk of your favourite wholemeal bread and you'll feel your halo shining with healthy goodness.

METHOD

1. Heat a small amount of olive oil in a pan (about 2 teaspoons).

2. Add onions and cook slowly over a medium heat. After a few minutes add garlic and soften with onions.

3. Add lentils, tomatoes, stock, coriander and spices to the pan and stir.

4. Bring to the boil and then simmer until lentils are tender.

5. Blend for a smooth consistency or leave chunky if you prefer.

Serve immediately with your favourite bread or chill for lunch at work the next day. Even if its pouring rain outside, this soup will put a little sunshine in your day. Leftovers can be frozen. ☺

(If you are suffering from heartburn, then this soup is just as good as a non-spicy version – simply miss out the turmeric and paprika).

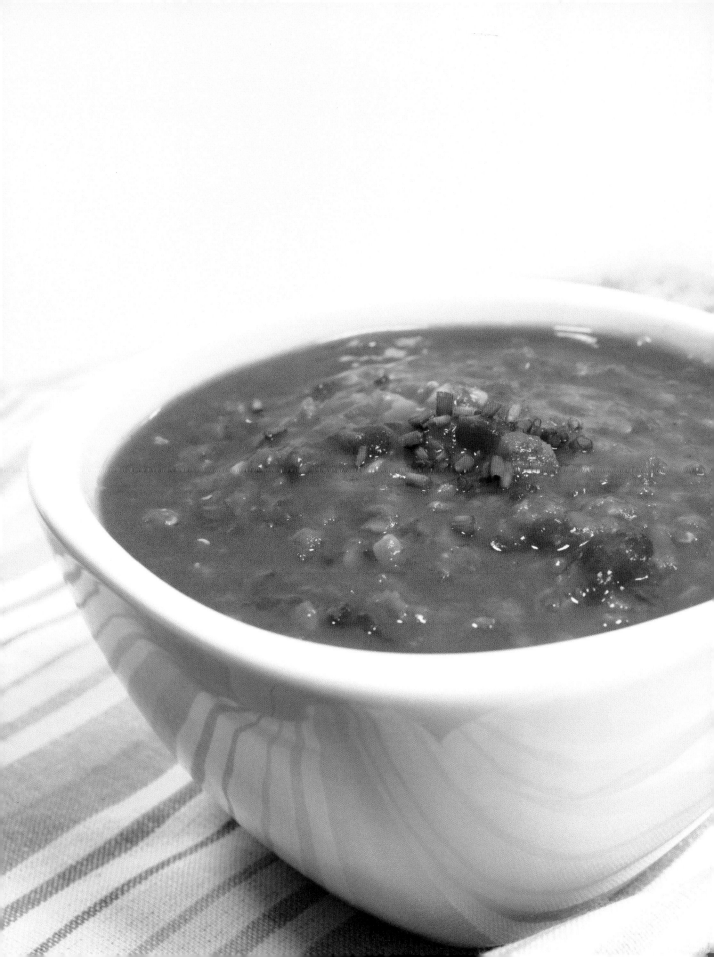

'Posh' ROAST BUTTERNUT SQUASH SOUP WITH ROSEMARY

INGREDIENTS

I large butternut squash or 2 small, peeled, deseeded and chopped

1 large onion, roughly chopped

2 garlic cloves, chopped

1 tablespoon honey

3 rosemary sprigs

750ml vegetable stock

2 tablespoons double cream

Juice of half a lemon

Serves 4
Preparation time 15 mins
Cooking time 40 mins

This is a posh soup and could be used to impress your friends and family at a dinner party. Why not have your own little private dinner party at work to treat yourself? The silky smooth creamy texture gives a hint of luxury which will see you rushing through your mornings work in anticipation. Remember you're worth it. ☺

METHOD

1. Preheat your oven to 200C (180C fan).

2. Put squash, onion and garlic in a large roasting tin. Add the honey and rosemary and mix well. Roast for 15 mins, take out and mix again. Return to the oven for another 15mins or until vegetables are soft.

3. Remove tin from oven and throw away rosemary.

4. Place roasted veg in a pot and add hot stock, bring to a gentle simmer. Ensure veg are fully cooked and then either puree with a hand blender or blitz in a food processor until soup is smooth.

5. Return soup to the pan and add cream and lemon juice. (If soup is very thick, add some water to your desired consistency). Season to taste and then warm through before serving.

If taking your soup to work, put a serving in a suitable container and chill overnight. Reheat at work and eat with your favourite bread. Show your colleagues your posh soup and make them jealous.

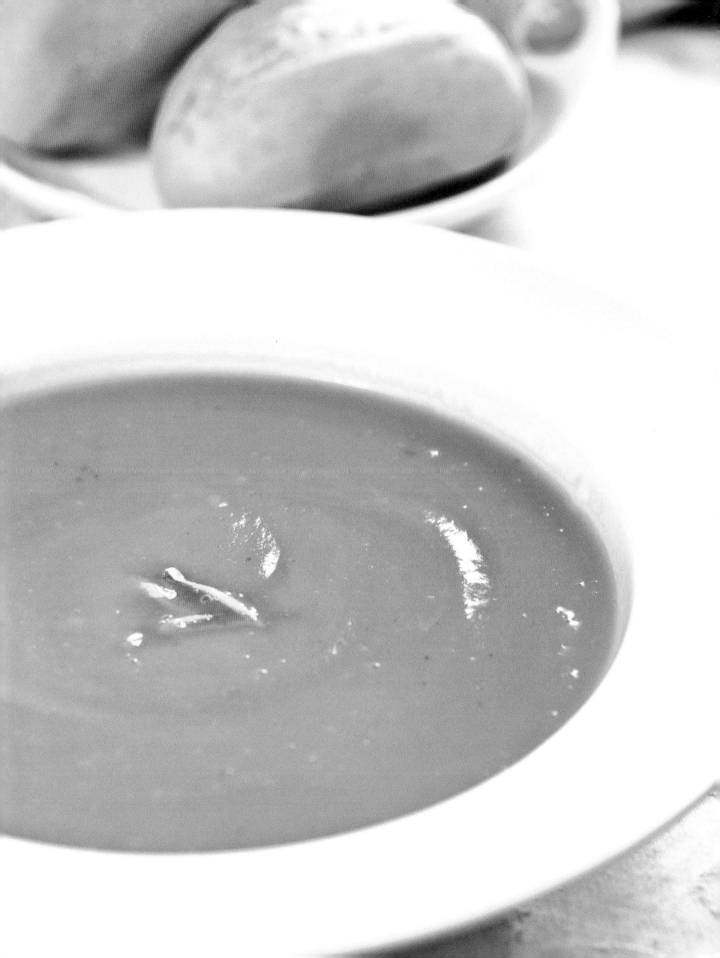

SMOKED MACKEREL PATE

INGREDIENTS

280g smoked mackerel fillets (about 1 pack)

200g cream cheese

Juice of half a lemon

1 teaspoon horseradish sauce (optional although gives a lovely flavour)

Oatcakes or wholemeal crackers to serve

Makes approx. 4 servings
Preparation time 10 mins

If you're not keen on oily fish or have never tried mackerel before, this super easy pate only takes minutes to prepare and is a great introduction to mackerel. The pate makes a good lunch or snack. Mackerel is a great source of Vitamin D, and omega 3 fatty acid. Vitamin D helps your body absorb calcium, which is needed for healthy bones and teeth. It is also made under your skin when you are outside in the summer months so if you are having a summer baby, sit outside to eat your lunch and get some extra Vitamin D!

METHOD

1. Remove the skin from the mackerel and discard. Break up the fillets and remove any obvious bones. (There should not be many).

2. Put the mackerel, cream cheese, lemon juice and horseradish in a food processor and whizz until all the ingredients are well combined. (You can use a fork to do this instead for a rougher pate).

3. Taste the pate for seasoning and then place in a serving dish.

Serve pate spread on the oatcakes or toast. Sliced red and yellow peppers eaten alongside go well for a great balanced dish.

(Only 2 portions of oily fish per week are recommended to keep a healthy balance).

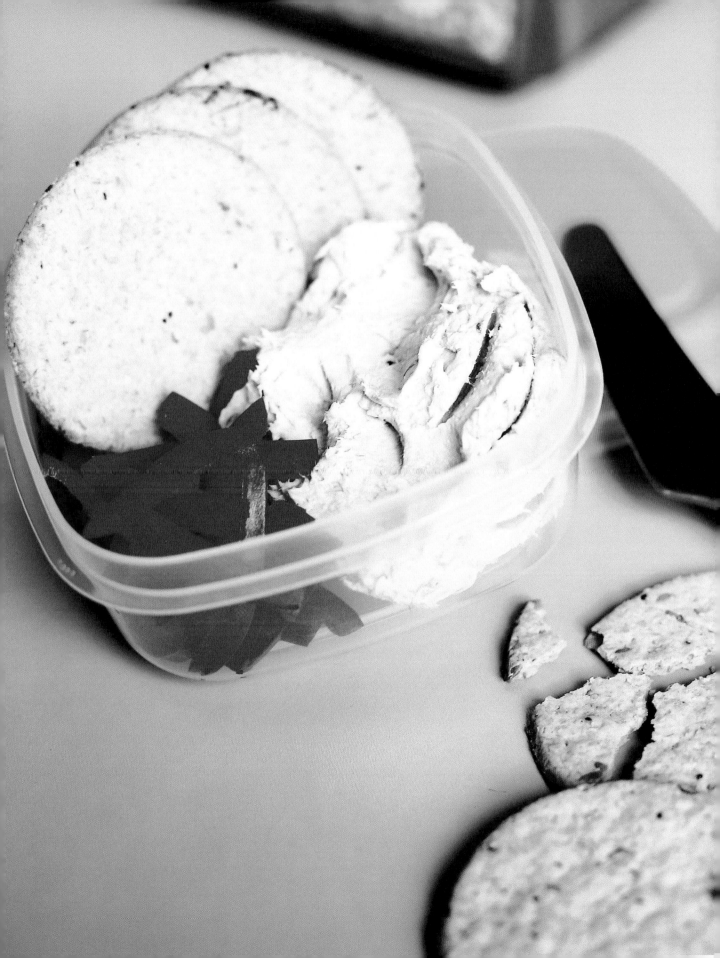

'Domestic goddess' FABULOUS FLAPJACKS WITH SEEDS

INGREDIENTS

175g butter

50g light brown sugar

140g syrup

200g oats (you may need up to 50g more depending on the brand of oats you are using)

50g mixed seeds (pumpkin, sunflower, linseeds, sesame or whatever you like)

Makes 16 squares
Preparation time 10 mins
Cooking time 30 mins

These will be a hit whenever you serve them and will last long in to your home baking future. Make some to take in to the office and impress your colleagues with your baking skills. Show them that you are an amazing baking mama. There is good news too. Oats are an excellent source of slow release energy and the seeds are full of essential fats. They don't just taste great but work hard for you too. When your energy levels start to drop, put your feet up (when your boss isn't looking) and enjoy one with a cup of tea. You know you deserve it. ☺

METHOD

1. Preheat over to 180C (160C fan).

2. Grease and line a 20cm square baking tin with parchment.

3. Place the seeds on a baking tray and toast in the oven for 5 mins or so. (Keep an eye on them as they burn easily).

4. Meanwhile place butter, sugar and syrup in a pan and melt over a low heat until simmering. Remove pan from heat.

5. Add oats in to the melted butter and syrup and mix well.

6. Add seeds and mix. If mixture is very wet, add more oats, spoon by spoon until the butter is soaked up.

7. Tip mixture in to baking tray and press down with the back of a spoon.

8. Bake for 20 to 25 mins until golden coloured.

9. Remove from oven and allow to cool for a few minutes. Mark in to squares before allowing flapjacks to cool completely.

Admire your baking and feel very pleased with yourself.

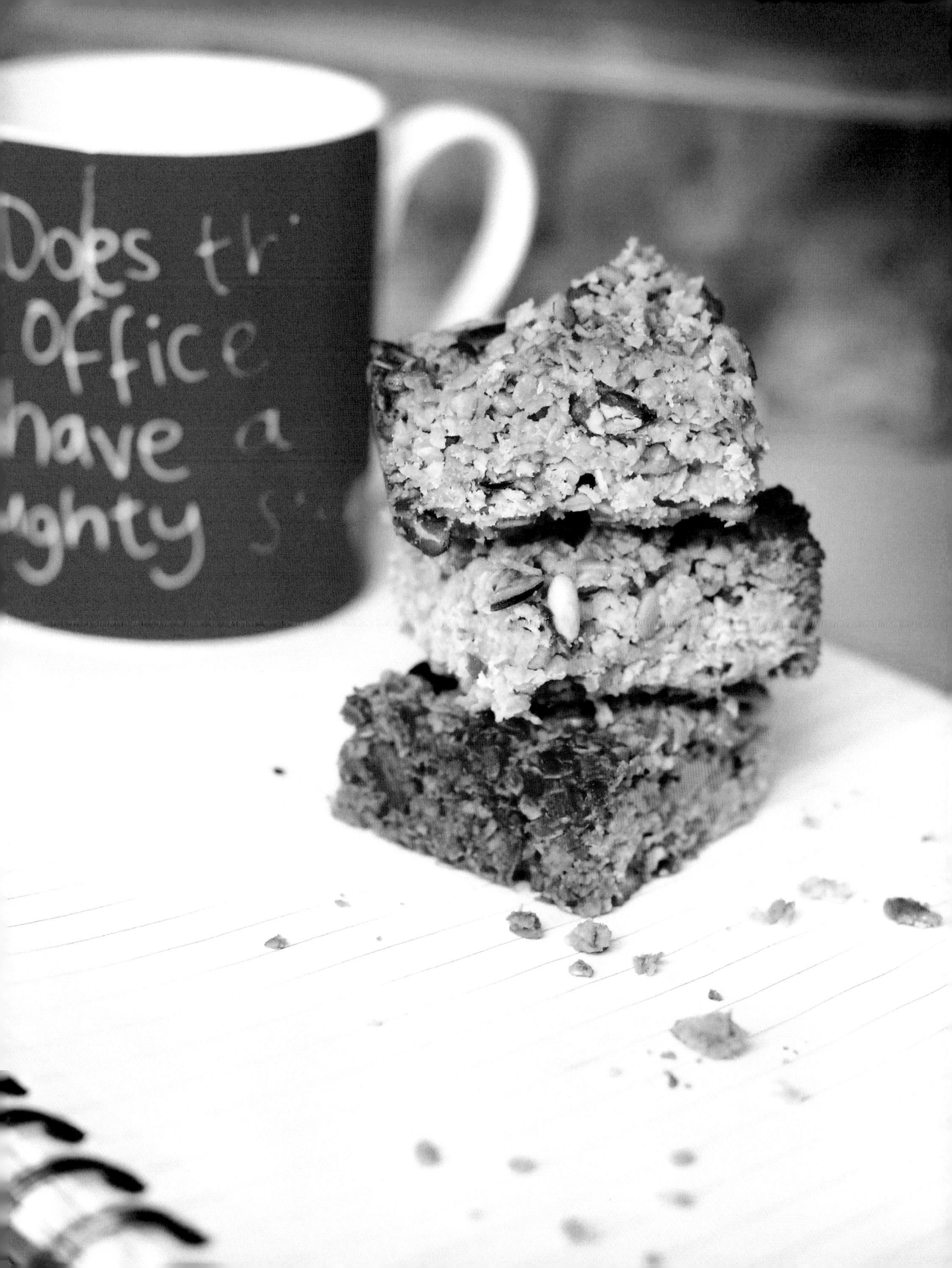
Does
office
have a

'I'm off on maternity leave'
BAKED LEMON CHEESECAKE

INGREDIENTS

250g digestives

125g butter

1 large lemon

500g cream cheese

142ml sour cream

2 eggs

175g caster sugar

1 teaspoon vanilla

1 level tablespoon cornflour

2 tablespoons sultanas (optional)

To serve, run a knife around the edge of the cheesecake and sit the tin on an upturned bowl. Gently release the side of the tin. Use a palette knife to loosen the bottom and slide cheesecake on to a serving plate (or suitable container for transporting to your work). Decorate with your reserved lemon slices.

When you are finished, take a moment to stand back and admire your cheesecake achievements. You truly are a domestic goddess. ☺

Well you've made it. You are nearly there and your last day is in sight. Maternity leave beckons and you want to leave your work with happy memories, happy colleagues and a great taste in your mouth. You can wow your work mates with this very impressive lemon cheesecake which is easy to make and tastes amazing. Take this in as a treat on your last day when work is nearly a distant memory. It should serve at least 12 people but you will need to stand guard as everyone will want seconds. (Note that cream cheese is safe in pregnancy and the eggs are fully cooked).

METHOD

1. Crush the biscuits in a food processor or put them in a sealed bag and crush with a rolling pin. Put biscuit crumbs in a bowl.

2. Melt the butter and add to the biscuits. Mix together.

3. Press the mixture in to a 20 cm round loose bottom tin.

4. Chill in the fridge for an hour.

5. Preheat oven to 180C (160C fan).

6. Grate the rind from the lemon and put aside. Halve the lemon and cut 3 nice slices from one half and put aside. (These slices will be used for decoration later). Squeeze the juice from the other half in to a small bowl.

7. Put the lemon rind, juice, cream cheese, sour cream, eggs, vanilla and cornflour in to a large bowl. Whisk together with an electric mixer until smooth. Stir in the sultanas if using.

8. Pour the mixture in to the chilled tin. Bake for 30 mins. Remove tin and carefully decorate with the lemon slices (pat them dry if very juicy). Return tin to oven and bake for another 10 to 15 mins until just set.

9. Turn off the oven and leave cheesecake inside with the door slightly open until oven cools down.

10. Put the cheesecake in the fridge until completely cold. Overnight is good.

Makes approximately 12 slices
Preparation time 30 mins plus chilling
Cooking time approx. 1 hour plus chilling

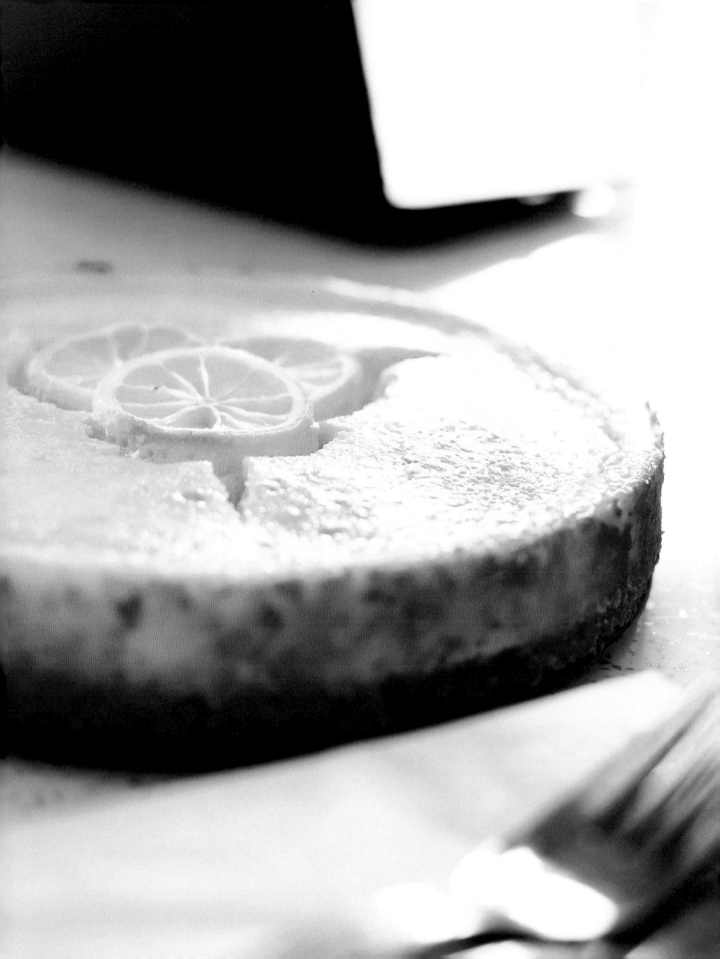

GOOD MOOD
Food

Crying in to your coffee at work for no reason? Welling up at the sight of a puppy or packet of newborn nappies? You are likely suffering from the normal emotional roller coaster of being pregnant. Looking after your emotional health is especially important in pregnancy as your moods can affect your developing baby. When you feel upbeat, positive, happy and calm, you produce hormones in your body which cross your placenta and give your baby these feelings too. The opposite is also true. If you feel sad or upset, your baby may experience this too so it's a good idea to be aware of your feelings and seek help if you experience a low mood which persists. The good news is there are lots of things you can do for yourself to keep pregnancy blues to a minimum. Start with the basics by making sure you are getting plenty sleep, exercising regularly and eating a good balanced diet. It's normal to have worries about labour, birth or becoming a parent, especially if this is your first baby. Talking to others who are at the same stage or have had children is really helpful. Learning breathing and relaxation techniques are great for your general wellbeing and will be very useful during labour, birth and as a parent of a new born too. If your low mood becomes persistent, you should always speak to your healthcare providers for additional help and support.

SALMON WITH PASTA
'and mojo'

INGREDIENTS

Olive oil

2 salmon fillets

2 slices prosciutto

200g asparagus, cut in to short lengths

150g pasta of your choice (fresh is quickest)

175g mixed peas, edamame beans and podded broad beans (frozen is fine)

5 tablespoons half fat mascarpone

Juice of half a lemon

1 tablespoon fresh tarragon, roughly chopped

Serves 2
Preparation time 5 mins
Cooking time 15 mins

This dish ticks a lot of boxes when it comes to healthy eating and the good news is that it tastes great too. Salmon is packed with omega-3 essential fatty acids which your brain needs to keep it working well. Also critical for the development of your baby's brain and eyes, salmon is an all-round winning choice.

Looking after your emotional health is particularly important during pregnancy when your moods can affect your baby's mood too. Choose to spend time with happy, positive people that you find easy to talk to and make you laugh. Get together for good food and a giggle and feed your mojo back. ☺

METHOD

1. Heat oven to 220C (200C fan).

2. Put your favourite funny movie on the TV while you cook or listen to some upbeat music.

3. Season the salmon and wrap a piece of prosciutto around each fillet.

4. Drizzle some olive oil in the bottom of a small roasting tin and lay in the salmon. Add the pieces of asparagus around and lightly toss in the oil.

5. Roast for 15 mins.

6. Meanwhile, boil the pasta according to packet instructions. Prepare your choice of pea and bean mix at the same time by adding to the pasta pan a few minutes before it is ready.

7. When the pasta and vegetables are just cooked, drain and reserve a cup of the cooking water.

8. Remove salmon from oven once it is cooked through and take it out of the roasting tin.

9. Add the pasta and beans to the roasting tin with the mascarpone, lemon juice and tarragon. Add a little of the reserved pasta cooking water to loosen the mixture to your preference. Mix gently.

To serve, divide the pasta between plates and place a piece of salmon on top.

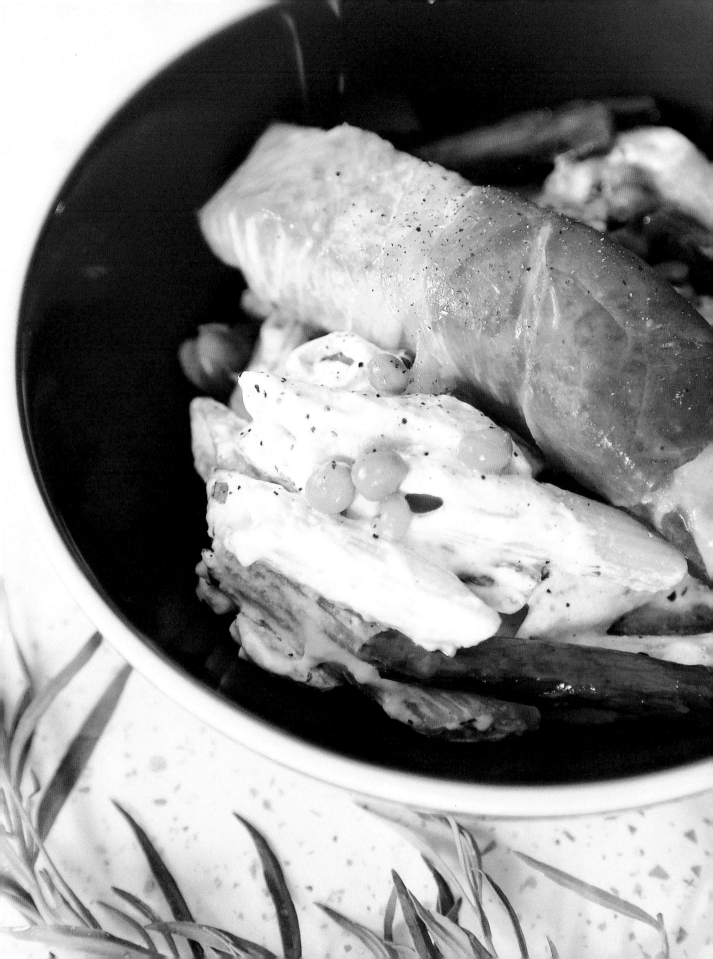

ASIAN STYLE BEEF AND NOODLE SALAD

INGREDIENTS

250 g lean beef mince

*1 red chilli, finely chopped or
1 teaspoon chilli puree*

1 clove garlic, crushed

50mls oyster sauce

Juice of a lime

150g bag cooked rice noodles

*1 carrot, peeled and cut
in to thin sticks*

*1 red pepper, cut in to
thin strips*

*Small bunch mint,
roughly chopped*

*I tablespoon unsalted peanuts,
roughly chopped (optional
although safe to eat in
pregnancy as long as you
don't have a nut allergy)*

Serves 2
Preparation time 10 mins
Cooking time 10 mins

Eating a rainbow of coloured fruit and vegetables every day means that you will get a good range of nutrients to keep you physically and mentally healthy. Lean beef contains protein which is needed for effective hormone and enzyme production, to support a good metabolism. This dish is also a particularly good supper to eat before or after exercising.

It is well known that exercise can improve your mood. This is due to the production of natural 'feel good' hormones produced as you work your muscles. Moving your body through swimming, dancing, yoga or walking are especially good forms of exercise in pregnancy. There is also evidence to suggest that women who exercise during pregnancy are more likely to have a normal birth. Plan to do a little exercise every day, even if it's just a walk to the local shop and you will be smiling all the way to the maternity ward.

METHOD

1. Dry fry the beef in a pan until browned all over.

2. Add the chopped chilli and garlic and cook for a few minutes.

3. Add the oyster sauce and lime juice and cook for a further 5 mins until sticky.

4. Warm the noodles according to pack instructions.

To serve, lay out 2 bowls and divide the noodles between each bowl. Top with the beef and then place a bunch of carrots sticks and peppers alongside. Add a few mint leaves and sprinkle with nuts, if using. Bon appetite!

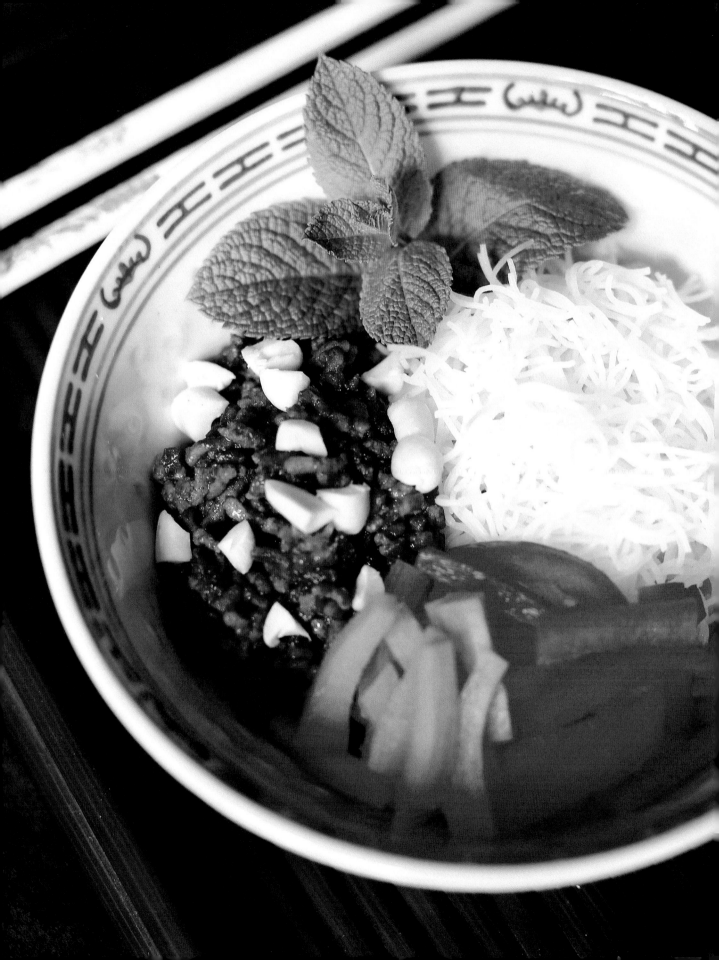

'Stress relieving'
CHOCOLATE SHORTBREAD

INGREDIENTS

250g butter, softened

175g caster sugar

200g chocolate (a mixture of good quality plain or milk chocolate works best)

225g plain flour

115g semolina

Makes 16 squares
Preparation time 10 mins
Cooking time 40 mins

This buttery shortbread is doubly delicious as it contains chunks of both milk and dark chocolate. Although unconfirmed, studies suggests that eating chocolate may reduce stress and produce happier babies! Even if it is not scientifically proven, eating some chocolate in pregnancy will certainly help make you smile. Need I say more? Get baking.

METHOD

1. Preheat the oven to 170C (150C fan).

2. Line a 20cm square baking tin with baking parchment or grease lightly with butter.

3. Put butter and sugar in a large bowl and beat either by hand or with a mixer until light and fluffy.

4. Stir in flour and semolina with a wooden spoon, then add the chocolate and mix gently. Don't over mix.

5. Put the shortbread mix in the prepared tin. Gently press down the surface and prick with a fork.

6. Bake for about 40 mins or until shortbread is a pale golden colour.

7. Take out of the oven and carefully mark out into squares after 5 mins. Allow to cool in the tin.

As a bakers privilege, you should eat a square of shortbread as soon as it is cool enough to handle.

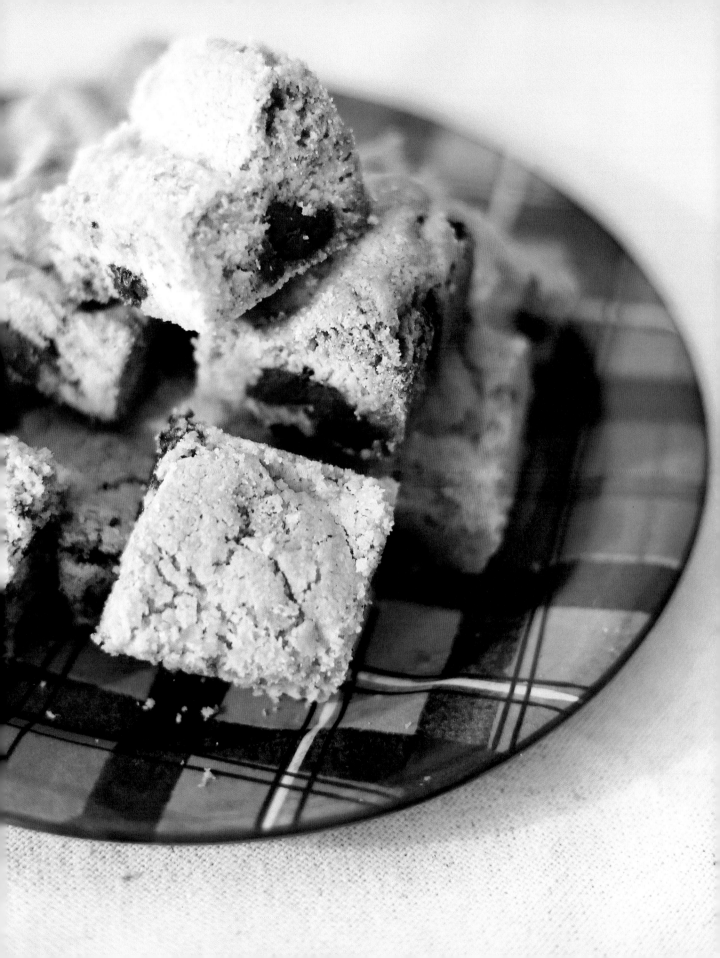

'Baby bonding'
DATE AND APPLE CAKE

INGREDIENTS

2 apples, finely chopped

155g chopped dates

Half a teaspoon bicarbonate of soda

250mls boiling water

185g butter, softened

220g caster sugar

1 egg

250g plain flour

Preparation time 15 mins
Cooking time 45 mins

Did you know that it is thought by some that your mood is connected to your digestive system and healthy hormone function? This might explain why you can feel content after eating a satisfying meal. This means that by keeping your gut healthy, you can also help your mood too. Constipation is a common issue for many women throughout pregnancy, and the early days after childbirth. This lovely cake is made with dates which contain a combination of soluble and insoluble dietary fibre which is helpful in promoting good gut transit. Help things along (☺) with a slice of this quick and easy date and apple cake and give your mood a lift too.

Take time out to sit down and relax while you eat. If you are on your own, put your feet up and spend a few minutes bonding with your bump. This doesn't mean using it as a shelf for your mug or plate (albeit extremely handy in the later stages of pregnancy), but it is about spending time talking to your unborn baby. Studies of newborn behaviour show that babies get used to voices they have heard in the womb and are more likely to respond to them once they are born. Try chatting, singing or reading out loud from a magazine or book and start to enjoy bonding with your baby today.

METHOD

1. Preheat the oven to 190C (170C fan).

2. Grease and line a 20cm square cake tin.

3. Combine dates, apples, soda and water in a bowl. Cover and leave to cool.

4. Cream butter and sugar in a bowl until light and fluffy.

5. Beat in the egg.

6. Gently stir in the flour and date mixture.

7. Pour in to the prepared pan and bake for about 45 mins.

8. Cake is ready when a cake tester comes out clean.

9. Allow to stand for 5 minutes before turning out on to a wire rack to cool.

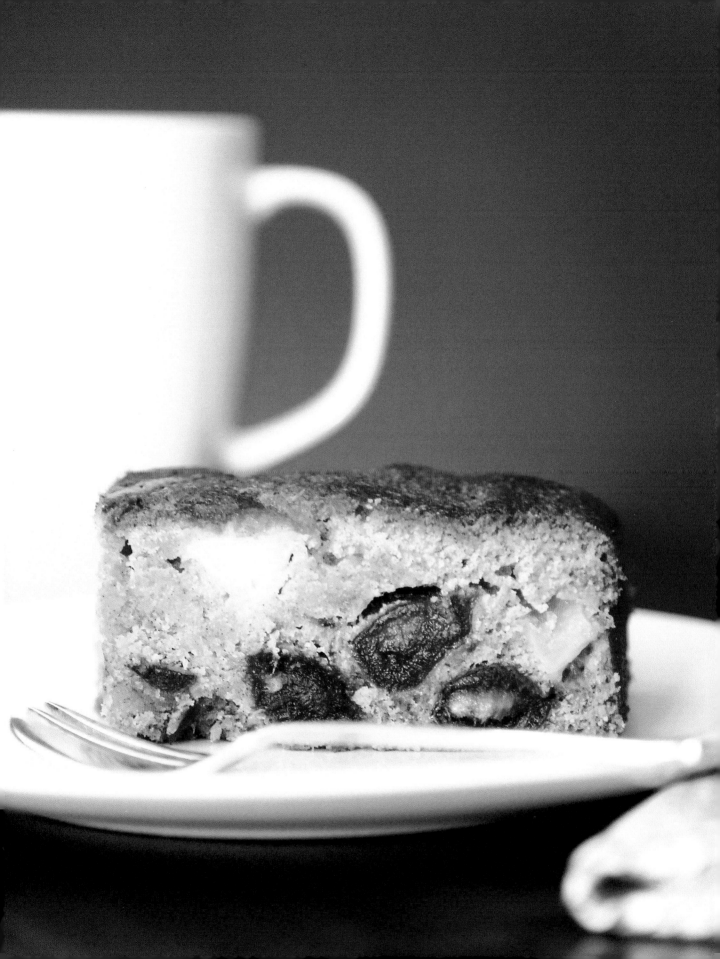

'Bedtime'
BANANA AND OAT SMOOTHIE

INGREDIENTS

2 tablespoons oats

5 tablespoons natural yoghurt

1 ripe banana, peeled

150mls milk

*1 teaspoon honey
(add more to taste)*

*Large pinch
ground cinnamon*

Serves 1
Preparation time 5 mins

This is a snack that packs a punch. The oats are full of fibre, B vitamins and iron. Oats also provide a slow release of energy which helps keep your blood sugar levels steady and avoids the swings in energy that can make you tired and irritable.   The yogurt is a perfect source of calcium which you and your baby need for bone health.

We all know that getting enough sleep helps to manage our mood. This can be tricky when you are up every 30 mins to use the bathroom or have a baby that likes to play 'kick the kidney' as soon as you get horizontal. If you are having trouble dropping off, learning breathing and relaxation techniques can be very helpful. There are many free apps which you can download or try the easy breathing technique at the end of this recipe. You could also make this smoothie as a mid-evening snack to stave off hunger pangs through the night.

METHOD

1. Place all ingredients in a blender and process until smooth.

2. Taste and add more honey if necessary

3. Serve over ice if you prefer your smoothie chilled.

Sit upright in your chair with your back supported or get comfortable in your bed. (Lie on your side in the recovery position with a pillow between your knees if your bump is big). Close your eyes and breathe in through your nose to a count of 5. Try to pull the breath deeply, down in to your tummy. Pause and then slowly breathe out through your mouth to a count of 5. As you breathe, focus your attention on your body. Become aware of any signs of muscle tension. (Starting at the top of your body and working your way down can help). During the outbreath, relax any tense areas. When you reach your toes, give your body a final check for any areas of tightness and then relax them. When you are ready, either gently open your eyes and have a stretch or allow yourself to drift off in to a lovely sleep. Goodnight. ☺

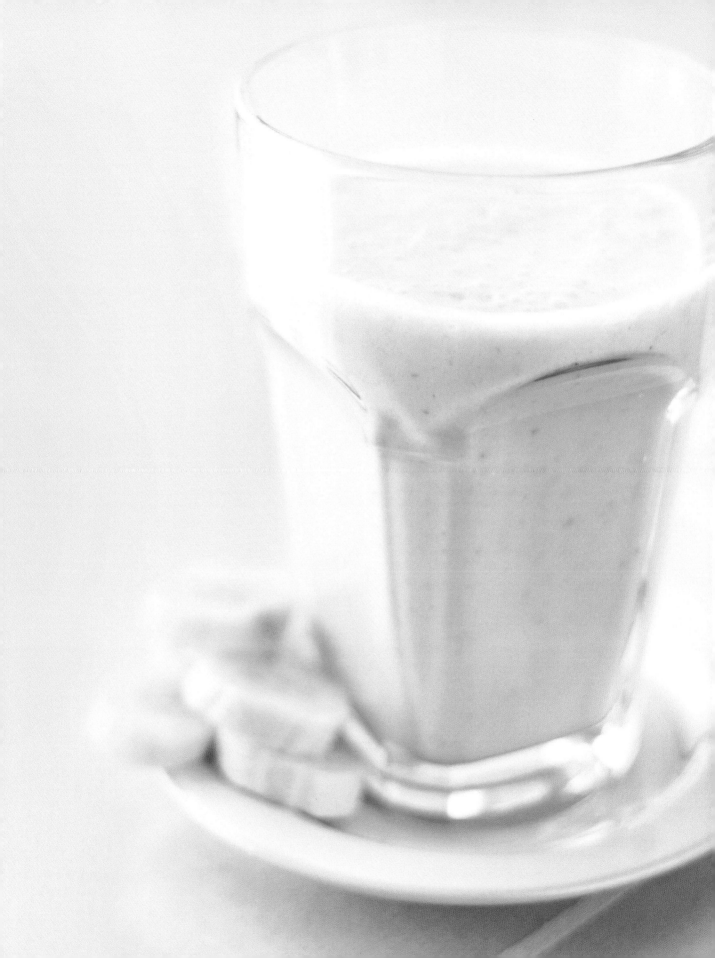

TEA WITH
Grandparents
TO BE

Whether your baby is the first grandchild in the family or the youngest in a long line, the news of a new addition always brings happiness and excitement. You may feel closer to your family than you have for a long time. Many expectant women (and men) find a new bond with their own mum and dad as they embark on becoming a parent. However, it is not unusual to become the subject of a lot of unwanted advice and well-meaning (but unhelpful) comments. Knowing that your mother hardly gained any weight when she was expecting you or that your mother in law did not get stretch marks is nice to know but not helpful while you are sitting on the sofa like a beached whale wondering if you will ever be able to tie your shoe laces again. (You will only understand this problem if you are at least 8 months pregnant).

Try to treat these comments as caring rather than letting them drive you crazy. You will probably need help and support when your baby arrives and your family are likely to be there for you first. Good communication is key. Have an honest chat now about the kind of help and advice you need rather than leave it until your baby arrives. Saying that you would prefer to ask for advice when you need it and learn from your own mistakes will earn you greater respect than having a tantrum every time your mum starts a sentence with 'when you were a baby we always/never'. It's a time of transition for everyone so make it easier by focusing on sharing your happiness and joy with the people you love.

'Good news' SLOW COOKED PULLED PORK WITH BAKED SWEET POTATOES

INGREDIENTS

1.5kg pork shoulder

1 teaspoon salt

2 teaspoon ground ginger

2 teaspoon ground cinnamon

1 and a half tablespoons dark brown sugar

4 sweet potatoes

Serves 6 plus leftovers
Preparation time 10 mins
Cooking time 5 and a
half hours including
resting time

Ready to announce to your family that you are expecting a baby? Want to make it a special event? Why not arrange a relaxed Saturday or Sunday late lunch and invite the important people in your life to join you. Even if you haven't managed to keep it a secret, it's still nice to plan a get together with your loved ones to celebrate that a new family member is on the way. Place this slow cooked pork on a board with the sweet potatoes around. Lay in the centre of the table and let everyone help themselves. Leftovers make a great filling for a wrap or sandwich.

METHOD

1. Preheat oven to 220C (200C fan).

2. Lay pork in large roasting tin and untie if it is rolled up with string.

3. Mix salt, spices and sugar together in a small bowl and then rub all over the pork.

4. Put pork in oven for 30 mins.

5. After 30 mins, remove tin from oven and pour 300mls hot water around the pork. Cover with foil. Reduce the oven temperature to 150C (130C fan) and return the pork to the oven.

6. Cook for 4.5 to 5 hours until the pork is tender, checking every hour and adding more water if necessary.

7. Meanwhile, wash the sweet potatoes and place on a baking dish. About 30 mins before the end of cooking time, add the potatoes to the oven.

8. Once pork is tender and pulling apart with a fork, remove the foil and increase the oven temperature to 220C (200C fan) for 10 mins. (You can leave the potatoes baking during this time if they are not ready. Test they are cooked with a knife).

9. Take out pork and leave to rest for at least 15 mins. Remove potatoes once they are soft.

To serve, lay the pork on a board and gently pull the meat apart with two forks. (You can leave some for people to do themselves if you want). Pour over a little of the cooking juices to keep meat moist. Serve the potatoes alongside with some steamed corn on the cob. Delicious.

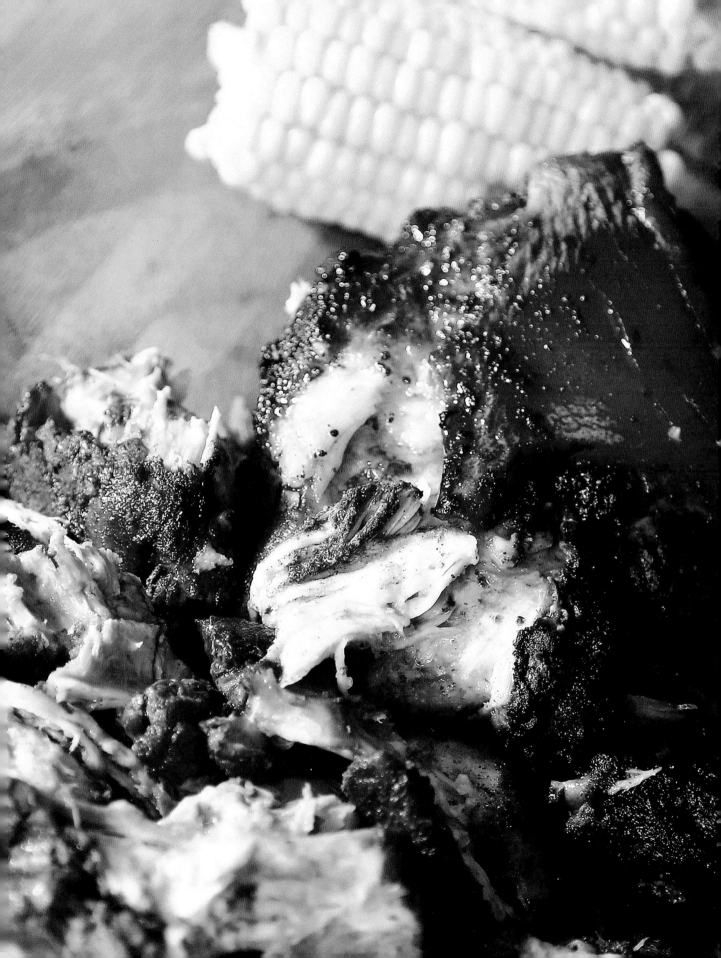

'Easy'
CHICKEN TRAY BAKE

INGREDIENTS

3 tablespoons tomato puree

3 tablespoons olive oil

1 red chilli, seeds removed and finely chopped or 1 teaspoon chilli paste

2 garlic cloves, crushed

8 skinless, boneless chicken thighs (approx. 600g)

500g small potatoes or large ones cut up

4 sprigs thyme

140g pancetta lardons

400g mixed tomatoes, cut up if large

Serves 4
Preparation time 15 mins
Cooking time 45 mins

Celebrate the start of your maternity leave with this tasty chicken dish. You can increase the quantity to serve a crowd so why not plan to have Mum and Dad and the outlaws over for lunch one day once you are off work? You are unlikely to have time to entertain for a while once your baby arrives so make the most of the last few days and weeks before the big event by building up favours with all potential future babysitters.

METHOD

1. Heat oven to 200C (180C fan).

2. Put the potatoes in to a pan of water and bring to the boil. Boil for 5 mins then drain.

3. Mix the oil, tomato puree, garlic, thyme and chilli in a bowl.

4. Lay chicken pieces and the parboiled potatoes in a large roasting tin and spread over the tomato and chilli mix. (Wash your hands thoroughly after touching the raw chicken).

5. Roast in the oven for 30 mins.

6. Remove tin from oven and stir in the pancetta and tomatoes. Return to the oven for another 15 mins until the potatoes and chicken are cooked through

Serve with a mix of vegetables such as sugar snap peas, green beans or mangetout.

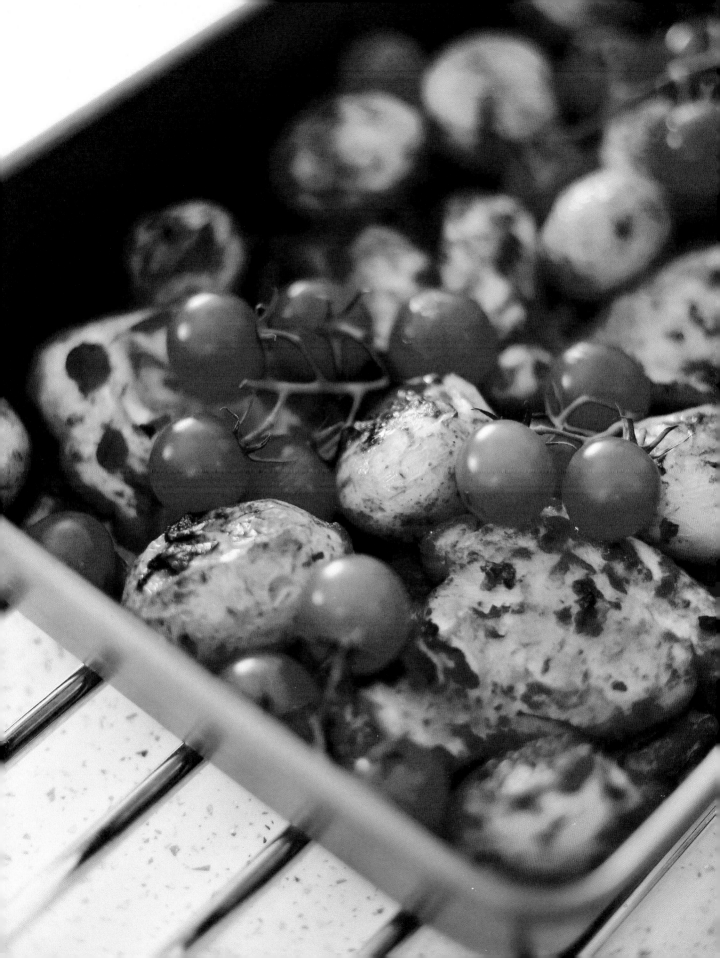

SALMON AND CHIVE BAGELS
'with mothers'

INGREDIENTS

*1 cooked salmon fillet
(about 100g)*

100g reduced fat cream cheese

Juice of half a lemon

*2 tablespoons fresh chives,
chopped*

2 bagels split in half

*2 small handfuls of
watercress*

Serves 2
Preparation time 5 mins
plus toasting time

Your mum has offered to take you shopping (and more importantly pay) for some baby stuff. Why not make a lovely lunch or afternoon tea for her to say thanks? This salmon mixture works just as well as a sandwich filler so choose what you prefer. Make the effort for your mum by setting out your nice cups and plates with a napkin. She will feel much appreciated and you will demonstrate you truly are the perfect daughter. (This would be a lovely treat for your partner's mother too).

METHOD

1. Remove any skin from the salmon and flake in to a bowl.

2. Add the cheese, lemon juice and chives.

3. Season to taste.

4. Gently mix together and refrigerate until required.

To serve, lightly toast the bagel and spread with the salmon mixture. Top with the watercress. Alternatively, thinly slice your favourite bread and top with salmon to make a delicious open sandwich.

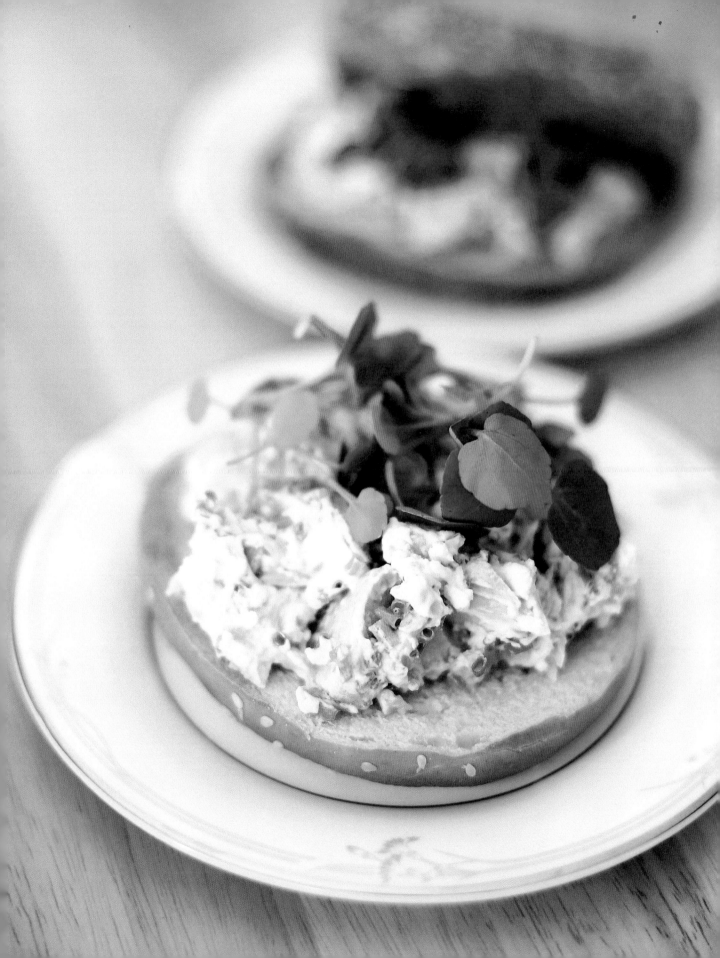

'Lazy Sunday' **RASPBERRY AND APPLE OATY CRUMBLE**

INGREDIENTS

4 cooking apples or similar, peeled and chopped

200g fresh or frozen raspberries

75g caster sugar

100g plain flour

75g oats

125g muscovado sugar

125g butter, diced

Serves 6
Preparation time 20 mins
Cooking time 50 mins

The combination of raspberries and apples in this scrumptious crumble is extra special. Save this pudding for the weekend as a treat after your Sunday lunch but be warned, you may need a nap afterwards. Don't feel too guilty though, as a portion must surely count as one of your five a day (well maybe).

METHOD

1. Preheat the oven to 190C (180C fan).

2. Put the apples and the caster sugar in a pan and cook gently for 5 mins until the apples begin to soften.

3. Meanwhile, place the oats, flour and sugar in a bowl. Rub in the butter until the mixture resembles breadcrumbs.

4. Put the apples in an oven proof dish (discard the cooking juice if there is a lot) and add the raspberries.

5. Tip the crumble mixture on top of the fruit and level off with the back of a spoon.

6. Bake for 40 to 45 minutes until golden on top.

Delicious served hot with custard, cream or vanilla ice cream. A small portion is enough. ☺

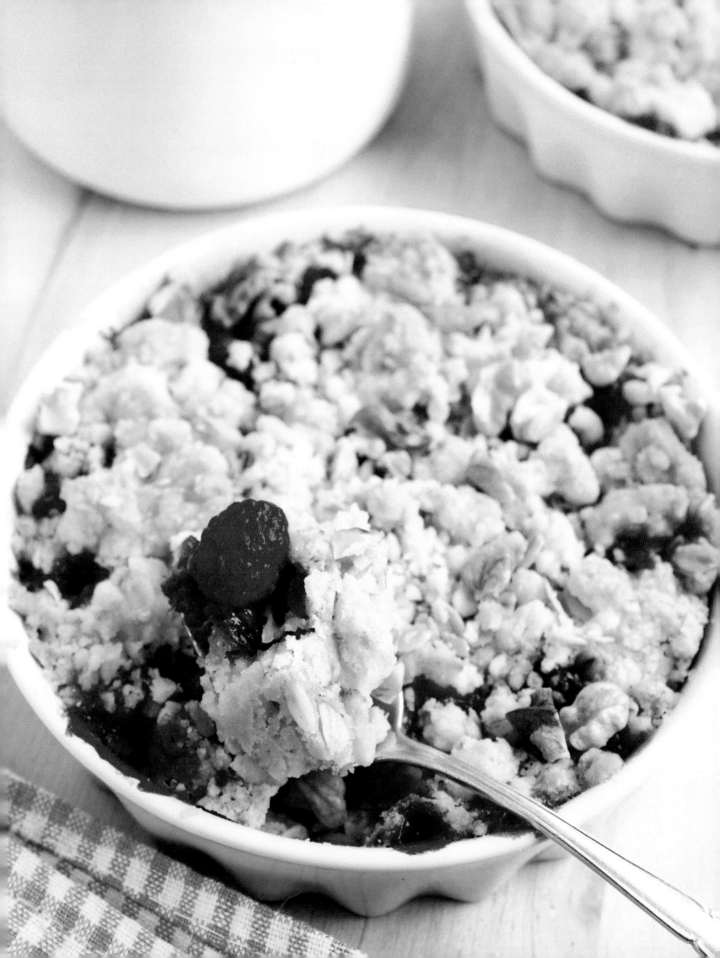

LEMON SYRUP CAKE

INGREDIENTS

125g butter, softened

175g caster sugar

2 eggs

Zest of 1 lemon

175g self-raising flour

4 tablespoons milk (approx.)

Juice of 1 lemon

100g icing sugar

Makes approx. 12 slices
Preparation time 20 mins
Cooking time 50 mins

This cake is sure to impress and is quick and easy to make. It's lovely served after the salmon and chive bagels as part of afternoon tea. Or why not wrap up some bagels and slices of cake and head off for a nice picnic at your favourite spot? You could invite your family along for an impromptu outing and spend an afternoon together enjoying the outdoors. Even if you are pregnant during winter, it is good to get fresh air, so wrap up warm and take a flask of hot tea. You'll definitely feel the benefit.

METHOD

1. Preheat oven to 180C (170C fan).

2. Line a 700g or 7cm x 21cm loaf tin with baking parchment (or use a ready shaped liner).

3. Using an electric hand mixer, cream the butter and muscovado sugar together.

4. Add the eggs one at a time and beat in between.

5. Add the flour and gently mix together with a wooden spoon.

6. Add the milk and mix together. (The mixture should be a soft dropping consistency. Add a little more milk if necessary).

7. Spoon cake mixture in to the tin and smooth the top. Bake in the oven for approximately 45 mins. A cake tester should come out clean when cake is ready.

8. While cake is baking, make the syrup by placing the juice and icing sugar in a small pan.

9. Heat gently until the sugar has dissolved then turn off the heat.

10. As soon as the cake is cooked and out of the oven, slowly spoon over the warm syrup, letting it soak in to the cake.

11. Leave the cake in the tin until all the syrup is soaked up and it is completely cold.

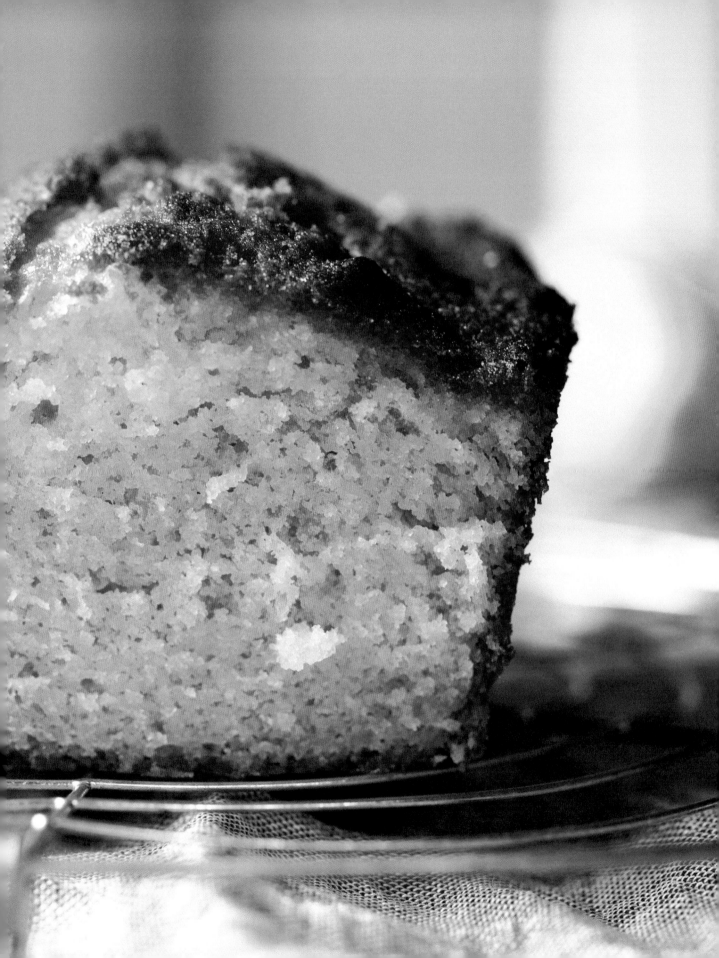

GOOD FRIENDS &

Get-togethers

Pregnancy provides a great opportunity to make friends and set up a new social network for yourself once your baby arrives. Being able to speak to others at the same stage of pregnancy is invaluable and can help reduce worry and stress. Antenatal classes are a good way to meet other women and your health professional can advise you of your class options. Pregnancy exercise courses such as aqua natal and yoga are also a great source of new friend potential. Check out your local area for bumps and babies groups too. Don't forget your old friends though. If they've had babies themselves, they will be a valuable source of knowledge and support. Why not plan some special dates with your girlfriends before your baby arrives? Do something you all love that also works for your stage of pregnancy and make some memories together. What about a pot luck lunch where you all bring a dish and enjoy sharing each other's favourite recipes? Sometimes friendships can get neglected once a baby arrives so make the most of your time together now and celebrate your friends.

– 68 –

SALMON WITH COUSCOUS AND
'other healthy stuff for you and your baby'

– 70 –

INDIAN STYLE CHICKEN WRAP
'with lycra'

– 72 –

'Time for dads'
STICKY BAKED SESAME CHICKEN

– 74 –

'Expectant mummy bonding'
BERRY CHEESECAKE

– 76 –

'BFF'
CHOCOLATE TRUFFLE CAKE

SALMON WITH COUSCOUS
'and other healthy stuff for you and your baby'

INGREDIENTS

100g broad beans, fresh or frozen (edamame beans also work well)

125g couscous

2 tablespoons olive oil

2 salmon fillets

Juice of one lemon

2 spring onions, finely sliced

1 tablespoon fresh mint, chopped

Serves 2
Preparation time 15 mins
Cooking time 20 mins

Growing a baby is an amazing event and sometimes it's hard to believe it's really happening. Although your first scan is an exciting milestone, feeling your baby kick for the first time is a moment you will never forget. Celebrate this extra special day with someone you love by eating a delicious supper filled with ingredients that even your baby will enjoy. You might get an extra kick!
Salmon is high in omega 3 fatty acids which has many benefits for your baby's growth including eye and brain development. Broad beans are rich in folate and other B vitamins needed for healthy nerves and blood cells.

METHOD

1. Cook the broad beans in boiling water for 5 to 10 minutes until just tender. Drain them and set aside. Once cool enough to touch, slip off their tough skins.

2. Put couscous in a bowl and pour over 150mls boiling water. Add 1 tablespoon of olive oil, stir and cover. Leave to stand for 10 minutes.

3. Season the salmon fillets with a little salt and pepper, then place on a tray suitable to go under the grill. Cook under a medium grill for around 5 minutes each side until salmon is cooked through.

4. Fluff up the couscous with a fork and then add the lemon juice, beans, sliced spring onion, mint and remaining olive oil.

To serve, gently flake the salmon and add to the couscous with the beans. Mix lightly together.

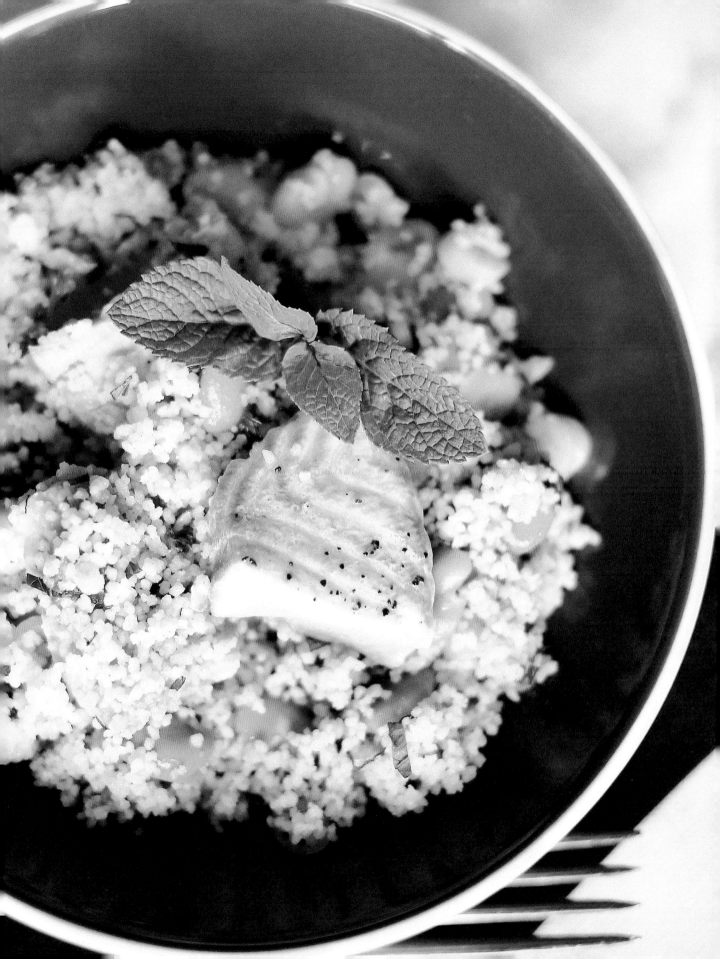

INDIAN STYLECHICKEN WRAPS *'with lycra'*

INGREDIENTS

150g low fat natural yoghurt

2 tablespoons hot curry paste

400g chicken thighs or breasts, boneless and skinless

Half a small cucumber, de-seeded and sliced

Half a red onion, thinly sliced

Juice of half a lemon

100g salad leaves such as baby spinach or lambs lettuce

100g low fat crème fraiche or natural yoghurt

1 tablespoon fresh mint, chopped

Wholemeal wraps to serve

Serves 4 small or
2 large portions
Preparation time 20 mins
Cooking time 20 mins

The day has arrived when you can no longer fit in to your favourite jeans and you know that maternity trousers are beckoning. How about a girls shopping trip to get you kitted out with your new pregnancy wardrobe? Let your hair down and breathe out at last. Enjoy lunch or supper together with these tasty wraps that won't add any more inches to your waistline.

METHOD

1. Mix the yoghurt and curry paste together in a bowl or dish big enough to fit chicken. Add chicken and mix well to coat. (You can use this right away or leave to marinade in the fridge for an hour or so).

2. In a separate bowl, mix the sliced cucumber with the onion and lemon juice. Set aside.

3. In another bowl, mix crème fraiche or yoghurt with mint and set aside. Put salad leaves in a dish to serve.

4. Heat the grill to medium and spread out coated chicken thighs on a clean tray. Place under the grill and cook for around 8 to 10 mins on each side or until chicken is cooked through.

5. Meantime, warm the wraps as per pack instructions.

6. Remove chicken and place on a board. Slice each thigh or breast in to bite size pieces.

To serve, place all the dishes on a board with the chicken. Lay everything out on the table and let everyone fill wraps to their taste. Enjoy.

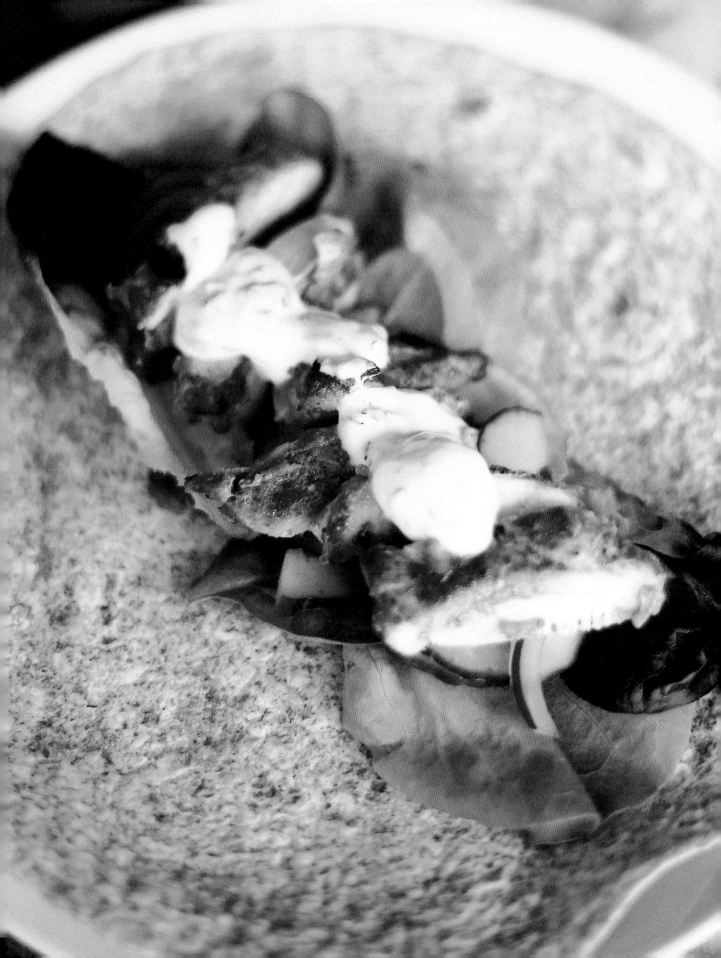

'Time for dads' STICKY BAKED SESAME CHICKEN

INGREDIENTS

600g chicken thighs, boneless and skinless

1 garlic clove, crushed

3cm chunk fresh root ginger, peeled and finely chopped or 2 teaspoons ginger puree

3 tablespoons orange marmalade

3 tablespoons dark soya sauce

1 tablespoon sesame seeds

Serves 4
Preparation time 5 mins
plus 15 mins to marinade.
Cooking time 35 – 40 mins

Okay, I know you are doing all the hard work growing a baby, but it's nice to celebrate your partner too. How about lunch with friends who are expecting (or have had babies recently) and their other halves? Sometimes partners don't get much chance to talk about having a baby with others at the same stage of the journey. A meal together as a group can provide an opportunity for everyone to air their views in a relaxed environment. This chicken dish is all made in one tray and can be prepared in advance so is easy for entertaining. You will get big brownie points from you partner and of course you can still get them to do the washing up.

METHOD

1. Mix the garlic, ginger, marmalade and soya sauce together in a large bowl.

2. Add the chicken thighs and mix to coat with the marinade.

3. Cover and leave in the fridge for at least 15 mins.

4. Preheat the oven to 220C (210C fan).

5. Lay the chicken thighs in a single layer in an oven proof dish and roast for 35 to 40 mins until cooked through.

6. Take the dish out of the oven and sprinkle over the sesame seeds. Return the dish to the oven for a few minutes to toast the seeds.

Serve with wholegrain rice, salad and a beautiful baby bump.

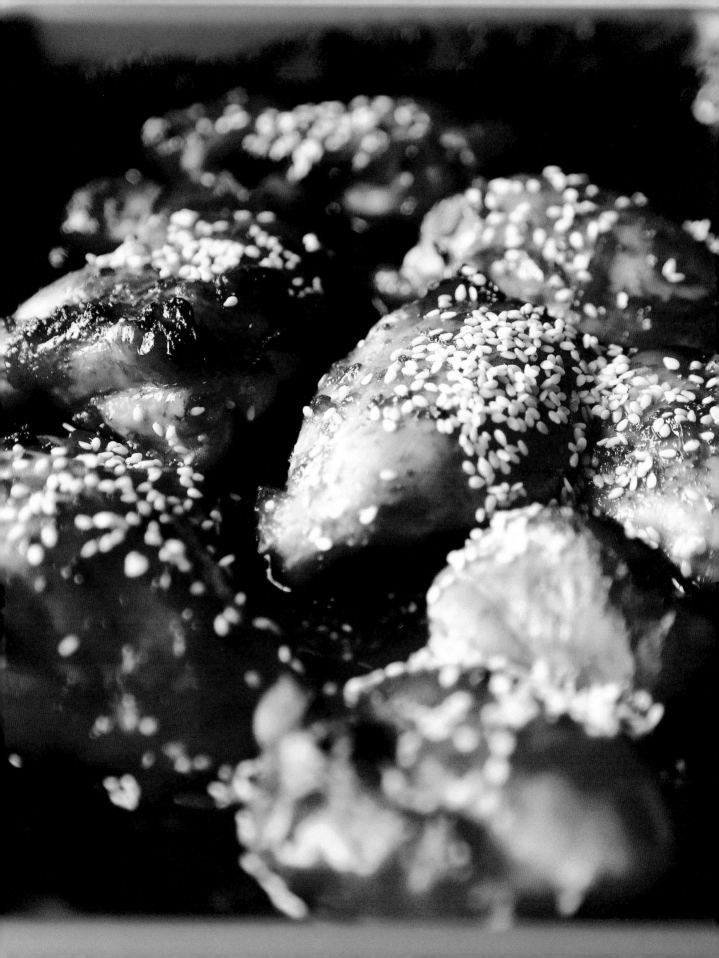

'Expectant mummy bonding'
BERRY CHEESECAKE

INGREDIENTS

10 oaty biscuits (such as Hobnobs)

250g cream cheese

Juice of an orange

75g caster sugar

3 tablespoons milk

142ml double cream

300g fresh raspberries

225g fresh straberries, stalks removed

Serves 4
Preparation time 20 mins

This easy cheesecake could also double as a very indulgent breakfast (for a special occasion)! It is a great recipe to enjoy with any new friends you've made through antenatal classes or other pregnancy related events. Getting together with people at a similar stage of pregnancy can create a great support network. Show your new friends you appreciate them by inviting them over for supper and treat them to this delicious 'expectant mummy bonding berry' dessert. Big hugs all round.

METHOD

1. Crush the biscuits by putting them in a sealed food bag and bashing with a rolling pin.

2. Put the cream cheese in a bowl with 50g of the sugar and the milk. Beat together until smooth.

3. In a separate bowl, whip the cream until it holds it shape. (Standing beating cream is a great time to practice your pelvic floor exercises. See point 6 in the celebration pancakes recipe for details). Gently mix the cream in to the cheese mixture.

4. Take about a quarter of the raspberries and strawberries and put in to a food processor. Add 3 tablespoons of the orange juice and the remaining 25g of caster sugar. Blitz to a puree. Pour the puree over the remaining raspberries and strawberries. (If you don't have a food processor, you can mash up the fruit, juice and sugar with a fork and then pass it through a sieve to take out big lumps).

5. To assemble, use a glass bowl or it can look very pretty in individual dishes - use four tumblers for this option.

6. Divide three quarters of the crushed biscuits between the tumblers or place in the base of the bowl. Spoon over half the fruit in the juice. Cover this with the cheese mixture. Top the cheese with the remaining biscuit crumbs and finish with the rest of the fruit.

This cheesecake is best assembled within an hour of eating.

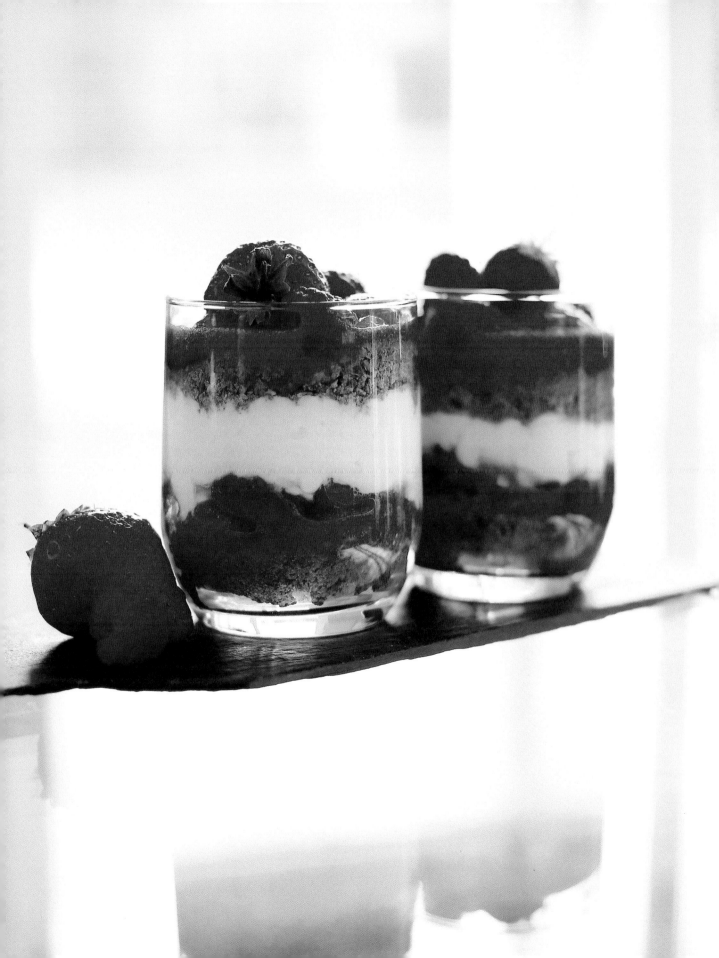

'BFF' DARK CHOCOLATE TRUFFLE CAKE

INGREDIENTS

1 tablespoon ground almonds

300g dark chocolate (min 60% cocoa) or 200g dark chocolate and 100g milk chocolate

250g caster sugar

165g butter

5 large eggs

Makes approx. 10 slices
Preparation time 10 mins
Cooking time 45 mins

This dense chocolate cake is good for any get together and even a small slice will satisfy most chocoholics. Lovely for a sophisticated coffee morning (decaff) or even better eaten warm with a scoop of ice cream, accompanied by your best friends, some good chat and your slippers.

METHOD

1. Preheat oven to 180C (170C fan) and butter a 20cm round loose bottom tin.

2. Break the chocolate in to pieces and place in a bowl with the butter and caster sugar.

3. Either melt over a pan of barely simmering water or melt in a microwave by cooking in 30 second bursts and stirring in between, until completely melted and combined. Set aside to cool slightly.

4. Whisk the eggs together with the ground almonds and fold in to the chocolate mixture. (The mixture will begin to thicken after a few minutes).

5. Pour chocolate mix in to the tin and bake for 35 to 40 minutes. (Mixture will still be slightly soft)

6. Allow cake to cool in the tin, then carefully remove to a plate.

Dust with cocoa or edible gold and serve with some crème fraiche on the side.

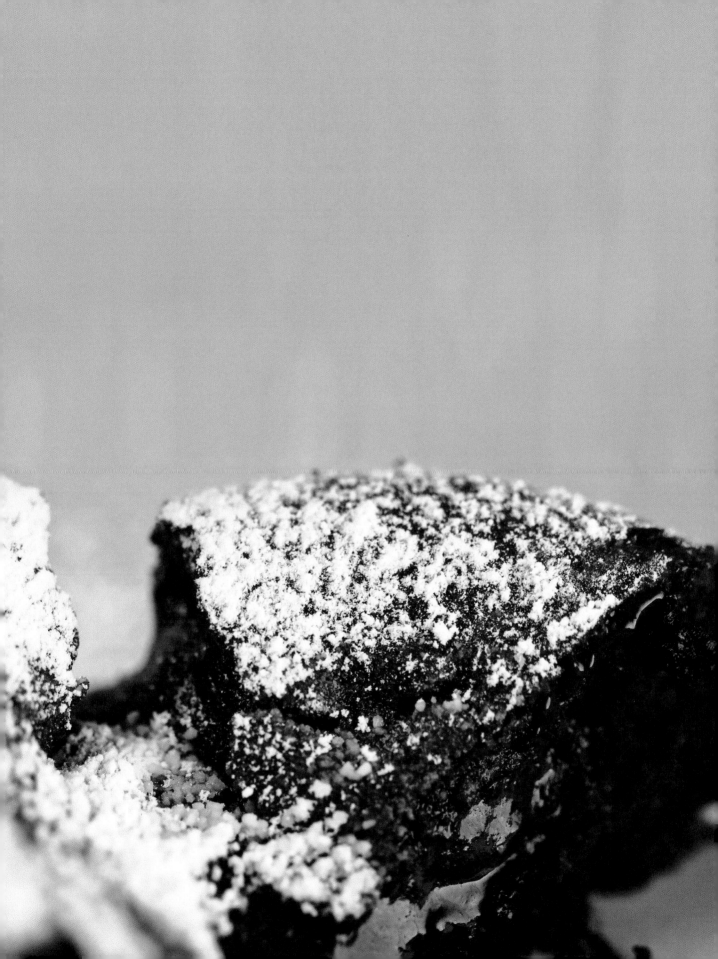

NAUGHTY
Nights In

You and your partner have made a baby together and are going to be parents. There is no greater achievement than bringing a brand new human being in to the world. You have the chance to celebrate this wonderful time together before your baby arrives so make the most of it and use every opportunity to be close and spoil each other. This is a time for closeness as well as having some fun. Pregnancy can make you feel very sexy or put you right off lovin'. Whether you feel like a damn hot mamma or you just need a cuddle and a foot rub, keep talking and be kind to each other. You'll be just great parents. ☺

– 80 –

'Baby bubbles'
MOCKTAIL

– 82 –

'Secret celebration'
STEAK WITH PASTA

– 84 –

'Baby nursery'
BARBECUE PORK RIBS WITH JACKET POTATOES

– 86 –

'Loved up'
CHICKEN KORMA

– 88 –

'Hand dipped'
CHOCOLATE COVERED STRAWBERRIES

'Baby bubbles'
MOCKTAIL

INGREDIENTS

50mls Pineapple juice

*125mls White grape juice
(such as Shloer)*

250mls Ginger ale

Makes 2 champagne flutes
Preparation time 5 mins

You may not have been a big drinker pre pregnancy or perhaps you enjoyed a few vinos on a Friday night, however, it is recommended that you give up alcohol for now. This can mean you sometimes feel a little left out at celebrations when everyone else is enjoying their favourite tipple. Baby bubbles mocktail is the answer. Don't miss out. Try this great tasting non-alcoholic cocktail to look like a grown up. You might never go back to the real stuff. Well maybe....

METHOD

1. Chill all the ingredients beforehand.

2. Mix everything together carefully in a jug.

3. Pour in to a cocktail glass or champagne flute.

Enjoy with a very naughty smile.

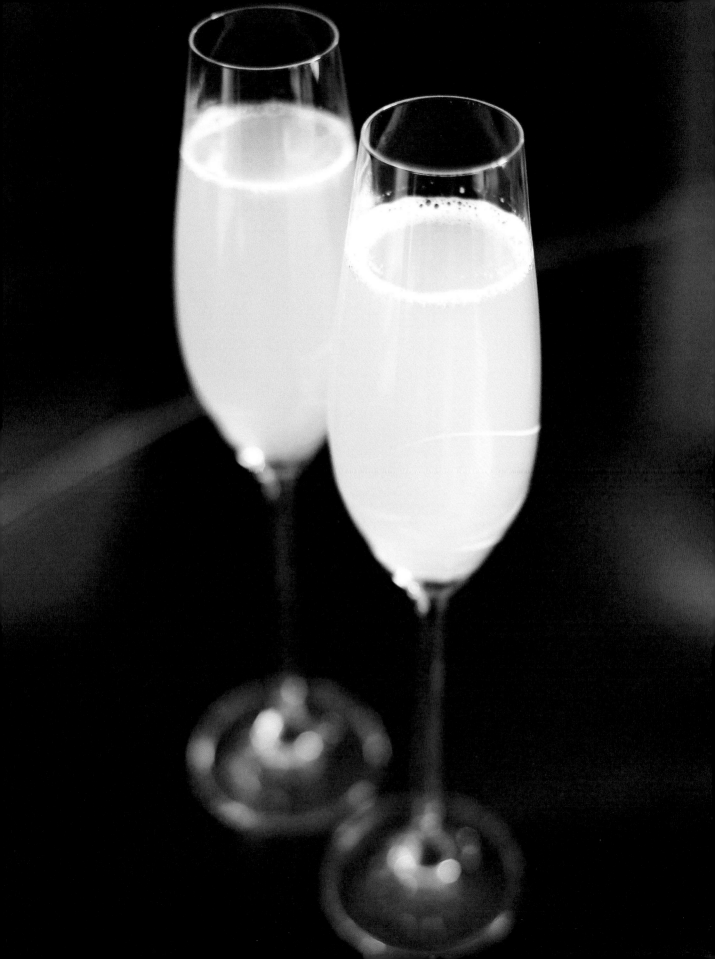

'Secret celebration'
STEAK AND PASTA

It's a unique moment in time when only you and your partner know you're pregnant. It's good to celebrate this special secret before you make your announcement to family and friends. A great way to celebrate is to have a really special dinner together. This quick and easy supper dish is just perfect for two. Make it really memorable by preparing your table in advance with your favourite dishes, napkins and candles. Choose some relaxing background music and put some flowers in a vase. Congratulate yourselves and make time to talk together about this super exciting time in your lives. Also, start off the evening with a Baby Bubbles Mocktail and make a special toast to each other!

INGREDIENTS

200g tagliatelle
(fresh is quickest)

1 teaspoon olive oil

(a little more may be required for frying)

1 x 200g sirloin steak

1 red onion thinly sliced

100g mushrooms sliced

100g half fat crème fraiche

1 -2 teaspoons Dijon mustard

Serves 2
Preparation time 10 mins
Cooking time 20 mins

METHOD

1. Put a pan of water on to boil for the tagliatelle.

2. Season the steak on both sides with salt and pepper and rub on the oil.

3. Heat a non-stick frying pan until it is hot, then fry the steak on both sides for about 3 mins each. (Steak should still be slightly pink inside but will get cooked again in the sauce). Remove the steak from the pan and set aside.

4. Add onions to the pan with little more oil if necessary. Gently fry until softened. Add a little water if they are sticking. This should take about 10 mins.

5. If using dried tagliatelle, put it on to cook now.

6. While the onions are cooking, remove any fat from the steak and thinly slice the meat in to strips.

7. Add the mushrooms to the onions in the pan and stir fry for a few minutes.

8. Pop fresh tagliatelle on to cook now.

9. Lower the heat in the frying pan and add the crème fraiche. Stir in 1 teaspoon of the mustard and taste. Add additional teaspoon if preferred.

10. Warm through for 1 to 2 mins then add the sliced steak and all the juices to the pan. Season to taste. (You can add some water here if the sauce is too thick).

11. Drain the pasta and add to the pan with the steak. Mix through, then serve on warmed plates.

Serve with a big smile and a loving kiss.

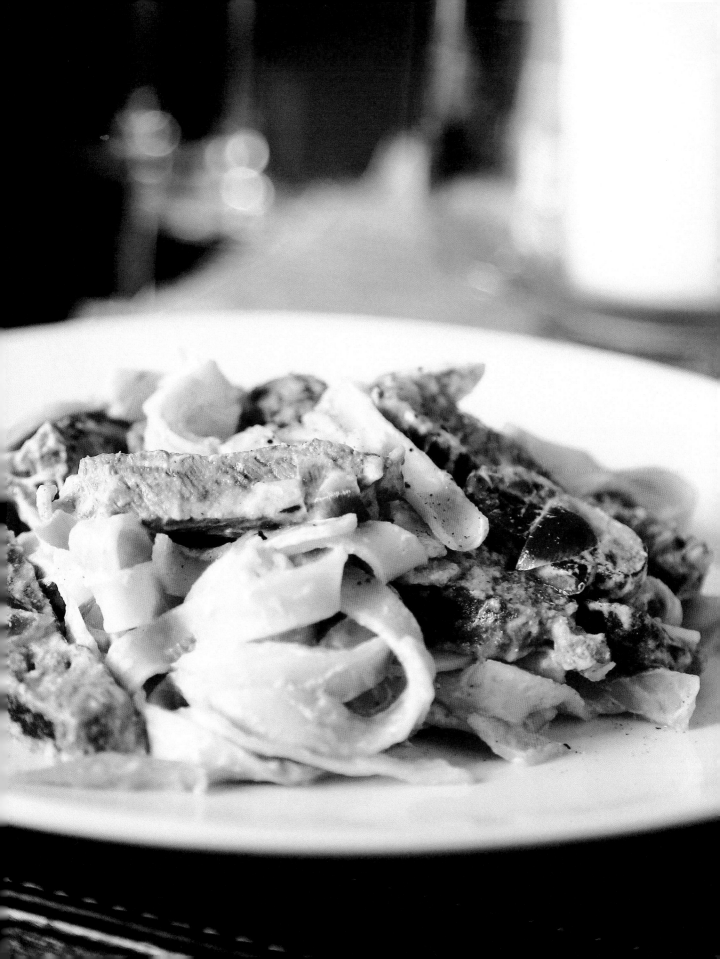

'Baby nursery' BARBECUE PORK RIBS WITH JACKET POTATOES

INGREDIENTS

500g pork ribs (in a rack or individual)

For the sauce

8 tablespoons tomato ketchup

4 tablespoons soft brown sugar

2 tablespoons Worcester sauce

2 tablespoons Soya sauce

2 tablespoons Sweet chilli sauce

1 teaspoon paprika

For the potatoes

2 large baking potatoes

2 teaspoons vegetable oil

Serves 2
Preparation time 15 mins
Cooking time 3 hours –
15 mins

Every movie about pregnancy seems to involve the exciting event of 'doing the nursery.' Although it is recommended that your baby spends its early months sleeping in your bedroom, he or she will eventually need a space of their own. Setting up the nursery is a very special project that you and your partner can enjoy together. While you get on with painting walls and putting together nursery furniture (or just supervising your partner doing these tasks), these lazy barbecue pork ribs can be slow cooking in the oven, ready for you to sit down and enjoy together after all your hard work.

METHOD

1. Heat oven to 160C (140C fan).

2. Lay ribs in a roasting tin in a single layer and cover with water. Cover tightly with foil and slow cook in the oven for 2 to 3 hours, turning once an hour.

3. Wash the potatoes and prick the skin with a sharp knife. Rub them with the oil and sprinkle the outside with salt. Lay the potatoes on an oven tray and cook alongside the ribs. (They will happily cook for as long as the ribs take).

4. Meanwhile, make the sauce by putting all the ingredients in a pan and heating gently until sugar has dissolved. Turn up the heat and allow the sauce to bubble for a couple of minutes before switching off.

5. Once ribs are cooked (meat should come away easily) remove from the tin and pour away cooking liquid. Return ribs to tin and coat all over with BBQ sauce. Remove jacket potatoes from the oven if they are cooked and keep warm.

6. You can store ribs in the fridge at this point if you want to keep them for later or immediately cook in a hot oven (220C or 200C fan) for 10 to 15 minutes until ribs are beginning to crisp at the edges. The ribs are also great barbecued.

Serve the ribs piled up on a board in the middle of your table with the jacket potatoes alongside. Coleslaw and salad both go well as accompaniments. Have a hug and cuddles for dessert. ☺

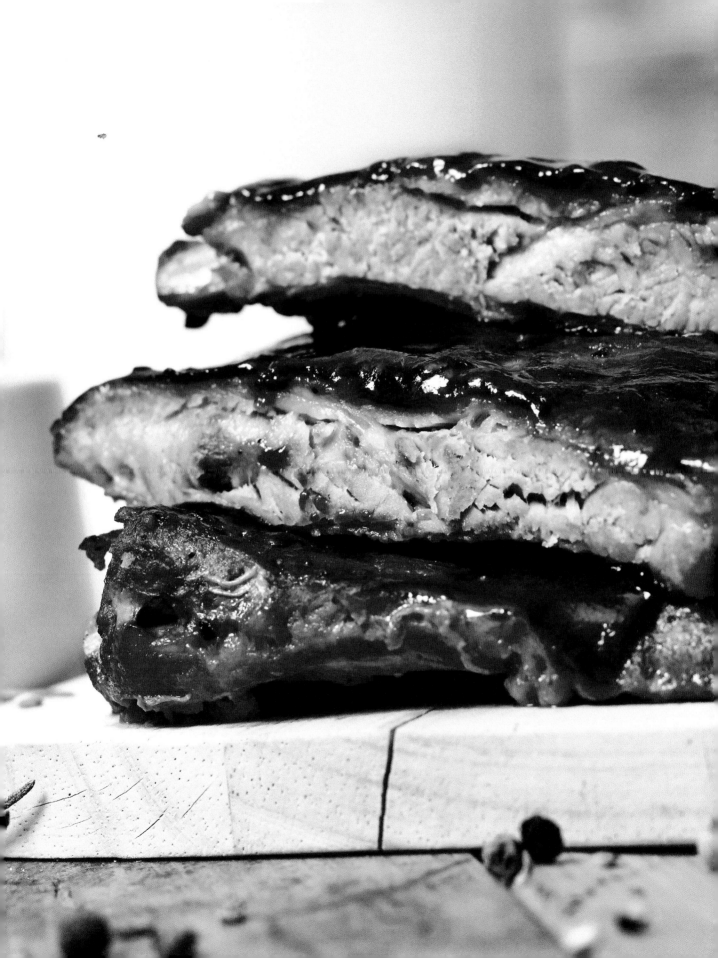

'Loved up'
CHICKEN KORMA

INGREDIENTS

1 onion, roughly chopped

1 garlic clove, peeled and chopped

1 thumb sized piece of fresh ginger, peeled and chopped

4 tablespoons korma paste

500g chicken thighs, boneless and skinless, cut in to pieces

2 tablespoons ground almonds

200mls chicken stock

Half teaspoon of sugar

2 tablespoons low fat Greek yoghurt

2 tablespoons fresh coriander, chopped

Serves 2 with 2 portions
for the freezer
Preparation time 10 mins
Cooking time 30 mins

Having a loving partner to share your journey to parenthood is such a wonderful thing. Soon you will have a third person joining your relationship who, no matter how wanted, will change things forever. Take every chance that you have to enjoy your last week's together as a couple. A holiday or night away before the birth can be very special or perhaps arrange a 'staycation' at home and plan some treats? Have a long relaxing bath together, spend the afternoon in bed, cuddle up and talk about your future as parents.

METHOD

1. Put the onion, ginger and garlic in a food processor and whizz to a paste. (Add some water if sticking).

2. Scrape the paste in to a high sided frying pan or wok. Add some water if you haven't already done so.

3. Cook paste over a medium heat for a few minutes.

4. Add the korma paste and cook for a further 2 minutes until fragrant.

5. Add the chopped chicken and stir before adding the almonds, sugar and stock.

6. Bring to a simmer and cook for 20 mins until chicken is cooked through. Add a little more water if korma gets very thick.

7. Switch off the heat and remove half to be chilled then frozen. Stir the yoghurt and coriander through the remaining korma.

Lovely served with brown basmati rice and naan bread in front of the telly watching your favourite romcom together.

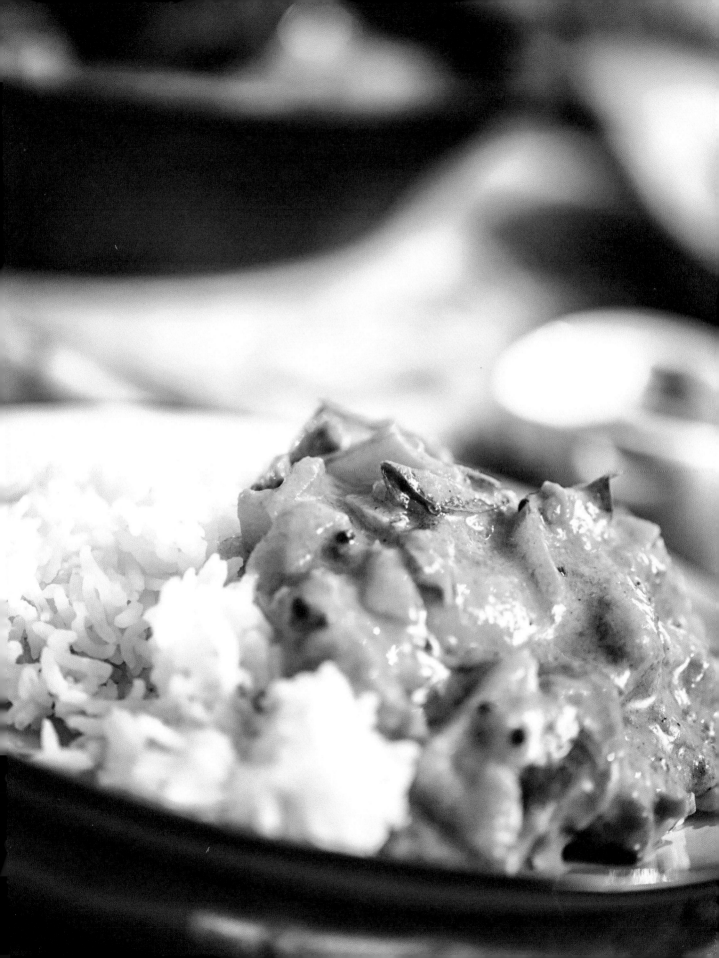

'Hand dipped' CHOCOLATE COVERED STRAWBERRIES

INGREDIENTS

1 punnet large strawberries with leaves

150g good quality chocolate (plain, white or milk)

Preparation time 10 mins
Melting time up to 3 mins depending on your microwave

Naughty but very nice. If romance is in the air, sharing these little treats with your partner can set the evening off nicely. Serve them as dessert or as an 'early night' snack – in or out of bed. If you are just not in the mood, eat them yourself in the knowledge that they still count as one of your five a day. ☺

METHOD

1. Rinse strawberries and pat dry. Lay out the best ones on a tray covered with baking parchment or tinfoil.

2. Break the chocolate in to small pieces and place in a microwaveable bowl.

3. Microwave the chocolate on full power for 30 seconds at a time, stirring in between until chocolate is fully melted and smooth.

4. Hold each berry by the stem and dip in to the chocolate, covering about three quarters of the fruit.

5. Return it to the baking parchment to set.

6. When all the strawberries are coated, place tray in a cool place to allow chocolate to fully harden. Avoid the fridge as it can discolour the chocolate (unless it is very warm in your home).

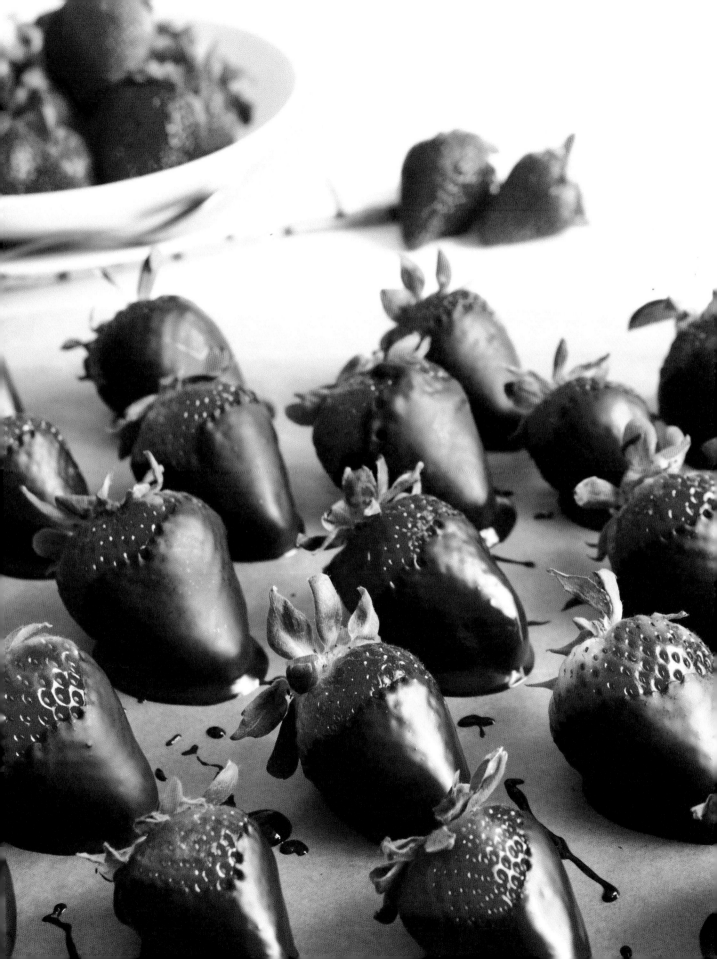

EMBRACE THE

Cravings

Thankfully due to our more balanced diets the time seems to have passed when pregnant women wanted to lick a piece of coal or nibble on soap. Nowadays, the most common cravings are for fruit, sugar, spicy or savoury foods. Ice is also surprisingly popular. Cravings can occur right through pregnancy although the first trimester is a common time when women's taste buds are affected by their changing hormones. Morning sickness can also make us crave one food and have a strong aversion to another. However there are still plenty of women out there who want pickles with their ice cream or who fancy ketchup on their custard! There is little evidence to prove why cravings happen. Have you already found yourself prowling about the house late at night, desperately craving something? Stay calm and try out these recipes. They have been chosen because they are very quick to assemble and satisfy the most frequent cravings in a flash or because they make a great snack which can be kept within reach at all times!

- 92 -

CITRUS FRUIT BREAKFAST BOWL

- 94 -

'Personalised'
FROZEN JUICE GRANITA

- 96 -

TOASTED PAPRIKA ALMONDS

- 98 -

'Sugar heaven'
APRICOT AND WHITE CHOCOLATE SQUARES

- 100 -

'I need chocolate'
TRUFFLES

CITRUS FRUIT BREAKFAST BOWL

INGREDIENTS

2 grapefruit (pink or red if possible)

2 oranges

2 passionfruit

60mls honey

90mls water

Makes 4 portions
Preparation time 15 mins
Cooking time 10 mins

Although slightly neglected as a fruit and not that fashionable, grapefruit is a great choice if you have a fruit craving. High in Vitamin C, lycopene and potassium, this citrus fruit brings many health benefits including having a positive effect on your blood pressure. The vitamin C helps your skin glow and helps keep your immune system on top form.

Enjoy this citrus feast for breakfast with a spoonful of natural or Greek yoghurt or eat as a snack at any time when you feel like a serious Vitamin C hit.

METHOD

1. Prepare the fruit by cutting the grapefruit and oranges in to segments. This can be done by first removing the skin and pith with a sharp knife. Then holding the peeled fruit in one hand, carefully slice down between the membrane of each segment with a knife. Remove each segment one at a time. (You may find a lot of juice comes off the fruit so catch it in a bowl and use this to replace the water in the syrup).

2. Combine honey, water (or reserved juice) in a pan. Bring to the boil and simmer gently for 5 mins. Remove from heat and cool.

3. Cut the passion fruit in half and remove the pulp.

4. Combine all the fruit in a bowl and pour over the cooled syrup.

5. Chill until required.

Eat on its own or serve with a dollop of Greek yoghurt.

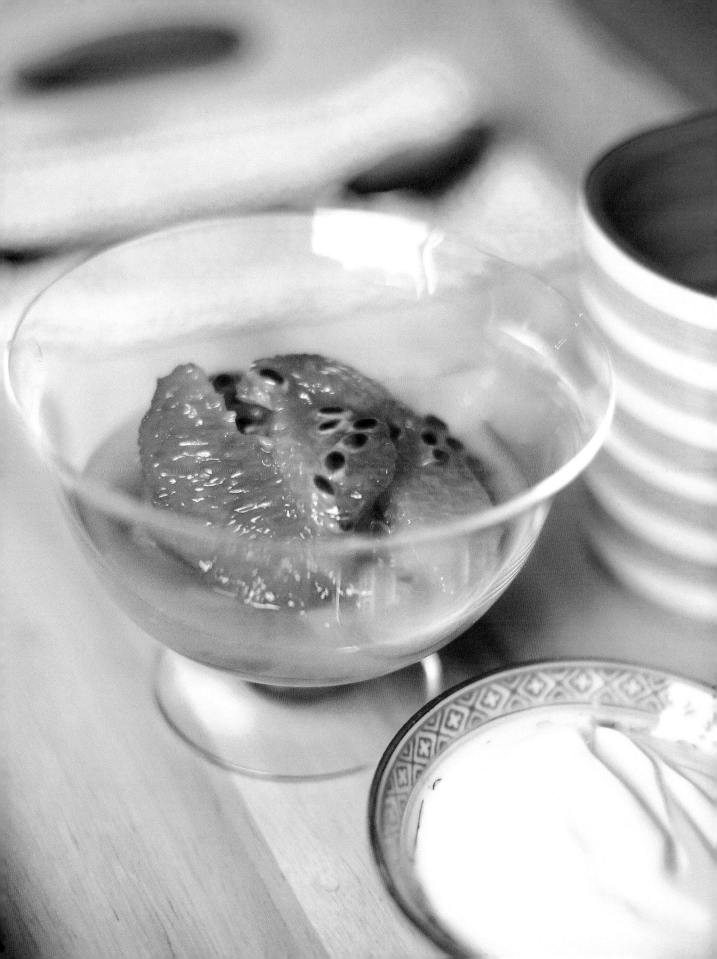

'Personalised'
FROZEN JUICE GRANITA

INGREDIENTS

200mls natural fruit juice of your choice

Preparation time 5 mins
plus freezing time

Who knew a day would arrive in your life when the prospect of sucking on crushed ice would seem appealing! This however is a common choice for many women right through pregnancy. Ice can be soothing in the early stages of pregnancy to alleviate nausea, it can cool you down on a warm summer day and is great to suck on during labour (when you just don't feel like eating).

By using your favourite natural fruit juice, you are also contributing a small token towards your five a day without adding too many calories! Keep some frozen cubes in your freezer so that you have them to hand whenever the need for crushed ice strikes. When you go in to labour, you could also consider taking some with you in a thermos flask – your own personal labour slushy.

METHOD

1. Fill an ice cube tray with the juice. (Silicon trays are easiest for ice cube removal).

2. Put in freezer and leave until completely frozen.

When a craving for ice hits, tip a few cubes in to a blender and crush to your preferred consistency. Alternatively, place a few cubes in a clean, sealable bag and bash the cubes with a rolling pin until you have your perfect slushy treat. ☺

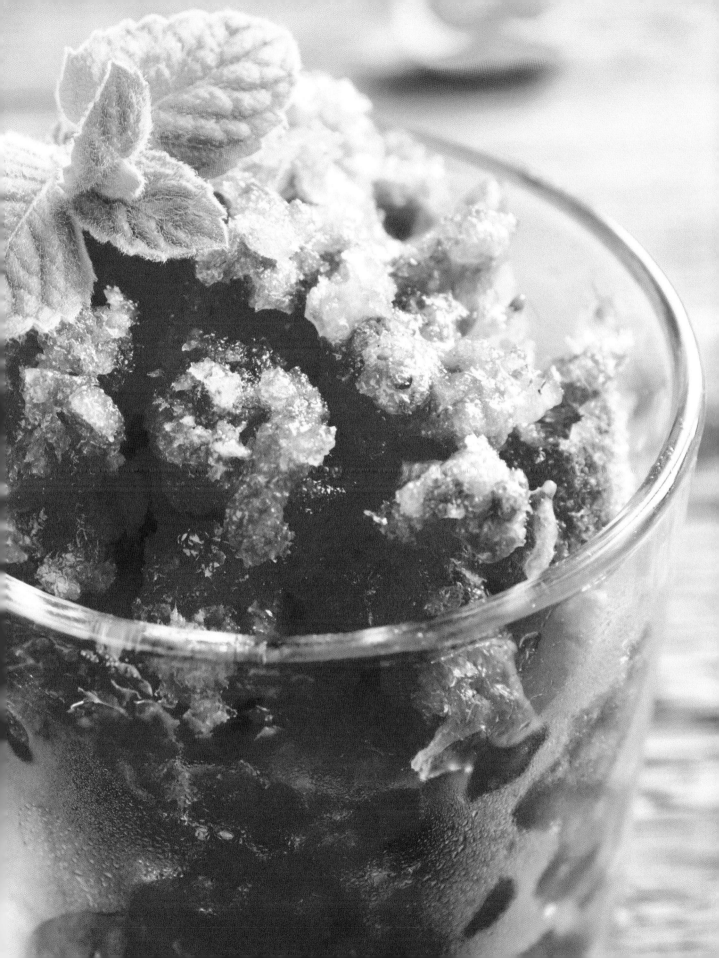

TOASTED PAPRIKA ALMONDS

INGREDIENTS

*300g natural almonds
(with skin on)*

Large knob of butter

1 teaspoon salt

1 teaspoon smoked paprika

Preparation time 5 mins
Cooking time 20 mins

Perfect to cure a craving for salty/spicy food, these toasted almonds are so easy to make and taste delicious. Great for snacking on, always keep a few in an airtight container for those moments when you just can't wait.

Almonds are a good source of protein which is essential for the healthy development of muscle in your growing baby. Your body needs protein for many things too. This includes preparing itself for the work of labour and birth so make sure you add a few to your diet and get yourself 'labour fit.'

METHOD

1. Preheat oven to 180C (160C fan).

2. Spread the nuts out on a baking trap and roast for 10 to 15 mins. (Keep an eye on them towards the end as they can burn easily).

3. Tip the nuts in to a bowl and add the butter, salt and paprika. Mix until the butter is melted and the nuts are all coated.

4. Pour the nuts back on to the baking tray and return to the oven for 2 minutes to dry the coating.

5. Store in an airtight container.

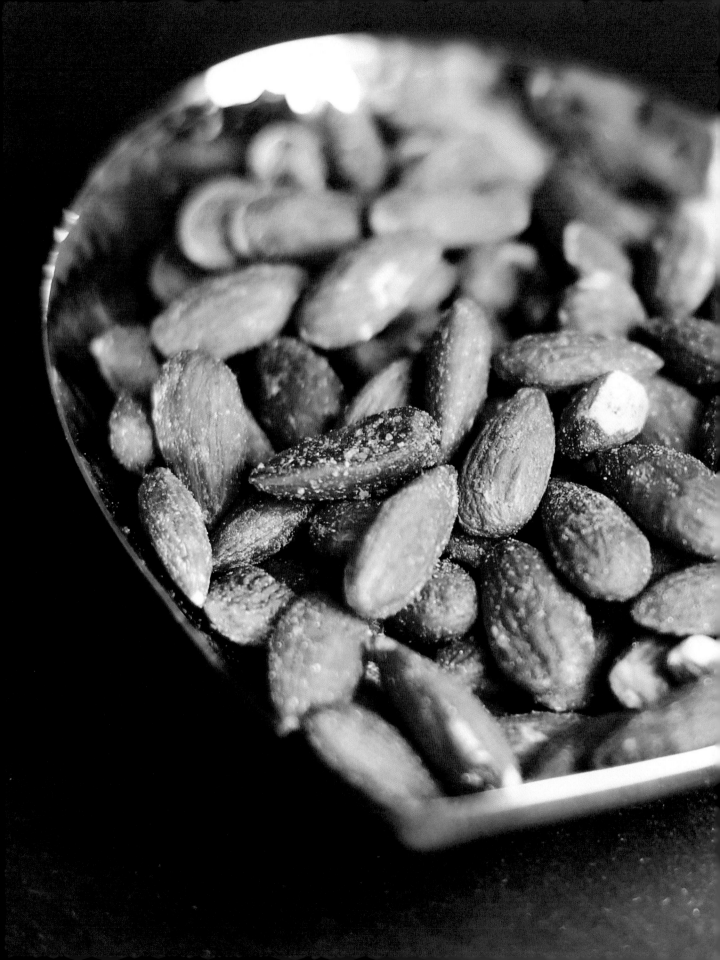

'Sugar heaven' APRICOT AND WHITE CHOCOLATE BARS

INGREDIENTS

150g oats

50g puffed rice

50g dried apricots, chopped

100g butter

85g golden syrup

75g white chocolate

Makes 16 squares
Preparation time 10 mins
Cooking time 10 mins
plus chilling time

These sweet crumbly bars are perfect when you need a sugar hit. White chocolate and golden syrup combine in sugar heaven. Don't panic though; apricots are considered one of your five a day so these cheeky treats are a mix of good and naughty. A craving for sugar could mean your blood sugar levels are getting low so try having healthy snacks between meals to avoid this happening. Of course, you may just have a sweet tooth and pregnancy is the perfect excuse to eat more treats! No one is perfect and there is nothing wrong with the odd sugar indulgence but alternate these with nutritional snacks to keep a healthy balance.

METHOD

1. Put the butter, golden syrup and white chocolate in a large saucepan and heat gently, stirring occasionally until melted together.

2. Remove from the heat and stir in the oats, crispies and apricots until well coated.

3. Press the mixture into a shallow 28 X 18 cm (11 X 7") lined tin.

4. Put in the fridge and cut in to bars when set.

Best stored and served straight from the fridge when the munchies hit.

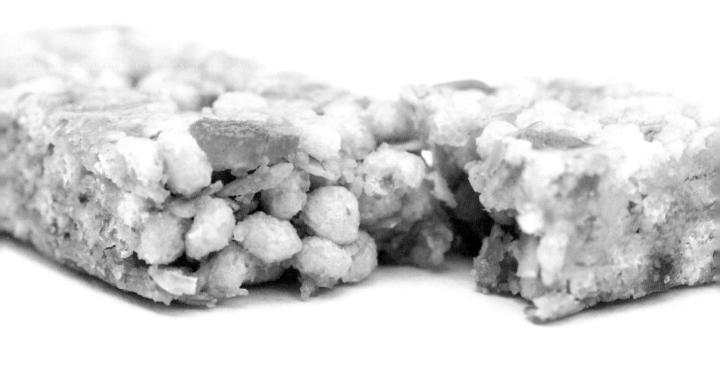

'I just need chocolate' TRUFFLES

INGREDIENTS

150ml double cream

1 teaspoon butter

150g good quality dark chocolate (min 70% cocoa solids)

Cocoa powder for dusting

Preparation time 10 mins
Cooking time 10 mins
plus chilling time

Sometimes we just need chocolate and nothing else will do. Pregnancy is a time when this craving may become overwhelming. You've seen the movies where partners head off to find an all-night supermarket (or in my case a 24 hour garage) to hunt down food for their chocolate deprived mate? Well, this unbelievably easy and truly divine recipe will keep those cravings at bay and reduce the need for late night foraging. They are so rich that one may well be enough (maybe). Keep a box in your fridge for those moments.

METHOD

1. Put the cream in a pan over a medium heat and warm until almost at boiling point.

2. Add the butter to the cream and stir to melt. Turn off the heat.

3. Chop the chocolate in to small pieces and put in a bowl.

4. Pour the warm cream over the chocolate and stir gently until all the chocolate has melted. (Add any alcohol at this point. A couple of teaspoons should be enough – see note).

5. Put the bowl in the fridge for a couple of hours until chocolate has set.

6. When set, remove from fridge. Sprinkle a tablespoon of cocoa on a tray or piece of baking parchment. Take teaspoons of the truffle mixture and roll quickly in to a rough ball in your hands. Roll the ball in the cocoa, then place on a plate.

7. Continue until all the mixture is used. (You may now lick your fingers and the bowl).

8. Store truffles in the fridge.

If you are going to share these with someone else (unlikely), you can split the mixture in two and add a little of your favourite alcohol to the non-pregnant portion. Liqueurs such as Cointreau or Grand Marnier work best.

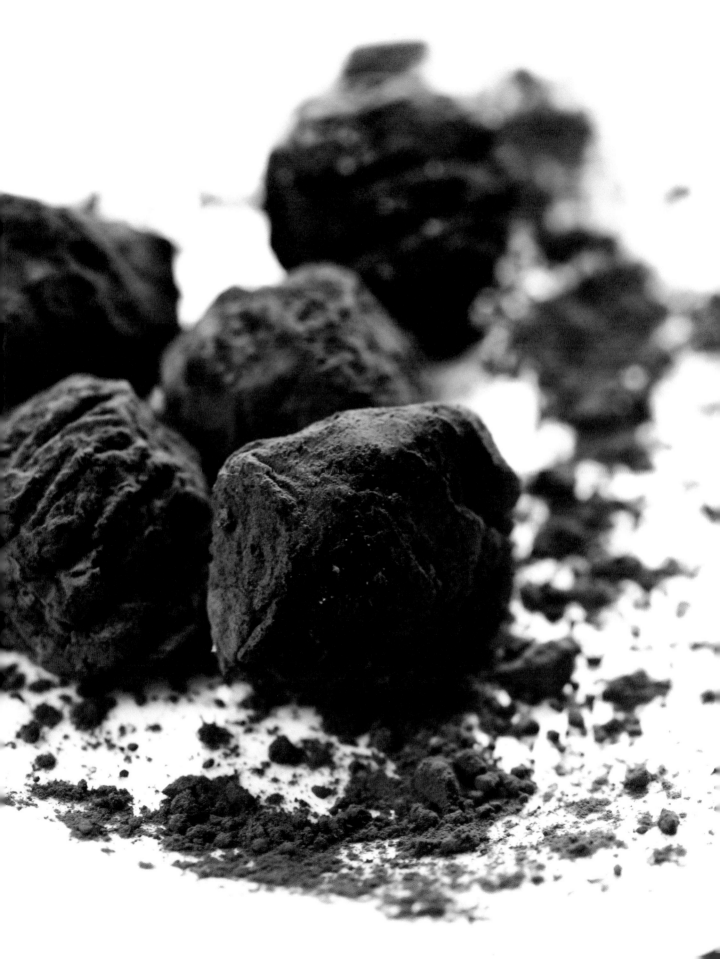

ABOUT THE AUTHOR

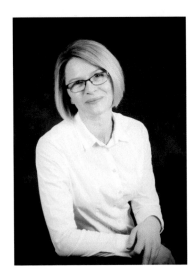

Emma has a diploma in antenatal education, a postgraduate diploma in HR and a degree in Biochemistry. She spent the early part of her career as an HR Advisor working in the energy industry. Following the birth of her third child, Emma trained as a childbirth educator and began teaching for the National Childbirth Trust. At the same time she was Director of The Baby Gurus Ltd, a company which provided support and education for expectant and new parents in the workplace. Emma published her first book 'Managing work and pregnancy successfully', in 2016.

Over the course of her work life, Emma has happily and successfully raised her two sons and daughter to adulthood, whilst living in Deeside, Scotland.

DISCLAIMER

The recommendations in this cook book are intended solely as information and should not be taken as medical advice. Please check with your health professional regarding your own circumstances if necessary.

ACKNOWLEDGEMENTS

A big thank you to everyone that helped me put this book together. Special mentions to Cameron Knott for his creative design work, Keilidh Ewen for her photography skills and Audrey McGregor (McGregor Dietetics) for her invaluable, nutritional advice and input. Also big thanks to my partner Steve for his encouragement, patience and good humour and to my son George for his recipe testing feedback.

12462123R00059

Printed in Great Britain
by Amazon